Faten LIMAIEM
Nadia BOUJELBENE
LEILA BOUHAJJA

Macroscopic examination in gynecology

Faten LIMAIEM
Nadia BOUJELBENE
LEILA BOUHAJJA

Macroscopic examination in gynecology

Essential protocols

ScienciaScripts

Imprint

Any brand names and product names mentioned in this book are subject to trademark, brand or patent protection and are trademarks or registered trademarks of their respective holders. The use of brand names, product names, common names, trade names, product descriptions etc. even without a particular marking in this work is in no way to be construed to mean that such names may be regarded as unrestricted in respect of trademark and brand protection legislation and could thus be used by anyone.

Cover image: www.ingimage.com

This book is a translation from the original published under ISBN 978-620-6-72674-6.

Publisher:
Sciencia Scripts
is a trademark of
Dodo Books Indian Ocean Ltd. and OmniScriptum S.R.L publishing group

120 High Road, East Finchley, London, N2 9ED, United Kingdom
Str. Armeneasca 28/1, office 1, Chisinau MD-2012, Republic of Moldova, Europe
Printed at: see last page
ISBN: 978-620-3-69490-1

MACROSCOPIC EXAMINATION IN GYNAECOLOGY
ESSENTIAL PROTOCOLS

TABLE OF CONTENTS

INTRODUCTION 4

TECHNICAL SHEET: FOETAL AUTOPSY 5

TECHNICAL SHEET: MACROSCOPIC MANAGEMENT OF
A MYOMECTOMY SPECIMEN 15

TECHNICAL SHEET: MACROSCOPIC MANAGEMENT OF
A SIMPLE ADNEXECTOMY SPECIMEN 21

TECHNICAL SHEET: MACROSCOPIC MANAGEMENT OF
AN OVARIAN CYSTECTOMY SPECIMEN 27

TECHNICAL SHEET: MACROSCOPIC EXAMINATION OF
A HYSTERECTOMY SPECIMEN 33

TECHNICAL SHEET: MACROSCOPIC MANAGEMENT OF
PLACENTAS IN TWIN PREGNANCIES 42

TECHNICAL SHEET: MACROSCOPIC MANAGEMENT OF
A CONE SECTION 57

TECHNICAL SHEET: PREPARATION OF CERVICO-
VAGINAL SMEAR SLIDES 61

RECOMMENDATIONS 68

CONCLUSION 69

REFERENCES 70

FOREWORD

In this invaluable compendium of protocols for the macroscopic management of gynaecological surgical specimens, we take a deep dive into the complex field of pathological anatomy. This book is a meticulous exploration of the essential details of macroscopy, offering an in-depth perspective on the examination of gynaecological tissues and organs.

As anatomopathologists and key players in the healthcare sector, mastering macroscopic protocols for gynaecological surgical specimens is of paramount importance. These protocols are the cornerstone of accurate diagnosis and effective management, with a direct impact on patient care and well-being.

This comprehensive manual is aimed specifically at professionals wishing to perfect their macroscopic skills and deepen their expertise in the analysis of gynaecological specimens. By exploring in detail the practical guidelines and methods specific to each type of specimen, it provides a comprehensive resource to support pathologists in their day-to-day practice. Ultimately, this guide aims to become an indispensable companion, offering clear protocols, relevant illustrations and practical advice for a methodical and rigorous approach to macroscopy in pathological anatomy, thus contributing to the continuous improvement of healthcare in the gynaecological field.

INTRODUCTION

At the heart of the fascinating practice of pathological anatomy lies the subtle art of macroscopic examination, a fundamental step that reveals the secrets hidden within surgical specimens. Each specimen, subjected to meticulous analysis including measurement, weight, palpation and dissection, reveals crucial clues to the underlying pathology. Guided by detailed diagrams and evocative photographs, pathologists embark on a captivating journey in which every element has a profound meaning.

Macroscopic examination is more than just observation; it shapes disease prognosis by identifying key parameters such as lesion size and location, influencing decisions about future microscopic analysis. From choosing which areas to sample to preserving specimens for further investigation, every step is essential to ensuring accurate and informed diagnoses. Fixation, a crucial stage, ensures the preservation of cell morphology and requires particular vigilance to guarantee reliable results. The precautions taken during fixation, such as the selection of the appropriate fixative, the size of the containers and the techniques adapted to the type of tissue, are essential links in the specimen processing chain.

Each phase of this meticulous process testifies to the unfailing commitment of anatomopathologists to unravelling the mysteries of pathology, offering invaluable keys to patient care and the advancement of medical research.

TECHNICAL SHEET: FOETAL AUTOPSY

Pathology Gynaecology

Educational objectives :

1) Methodically carry out a foetal dissection, referring to an index card.
technique.
2) When dissecting the foetus, take the samples required for the following tests
further tests.
3) Identify any congenital anomalies during foetal dissection.

INTRODUCTION

Foetal autopsy is an increasingly common examination. It may be requested in the event of
miscarriage, medical termination of pregnancy or foetal death in utero. It completes the
assessment of a pathological pregnancy and is an essential part of **genetic counselling.**
Fetal autopsy is a key stage in the multidisciplinary management of a pathological pregnancy
It is carried out according to local availability and agreements between different teams.

MATERIAL REQUIRED

1. Flexible tape measure for circumferences
2. Graduated rulers
3. Calipers for diameters
4. A knife
5. A scalpel with its blade
6. Pliers with and without claws
7. Probes, including an olive-tip probe
8. Foam-tipped scissors
9. Cassettes
10. Camera

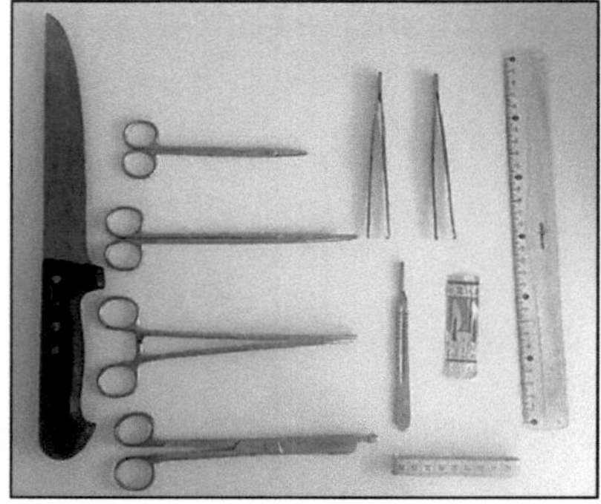

Figure 1: Dissecting equipment used during foetal autopsy.

Special sampling equipment :

1. Culture medium for karyotype
2. Freezer tubes
3. Sterile tubes and jars for bacteriological studies
4. Sterile syringes and needles

METHODOLOGY

• The foetopathological examination involves several successive stages which must be carried out in a given order in order to ensure the quality of the examination.

• Photographs are taken systematically. They are essential for documenting malformations.

A. EXTERNAL EXAMINATION

• The state of **maceration** of the foetus is assessed.

• A macerated foetus is a sign of foetal death in utero.

• Maceration results in hypotonia, epidermolysis (skin detachment), a reddish-brown colour of the foetus, a vinous colouration of the cord and overlapping of the skull bones.

• If the retention period is very long, **mummification** may occur.

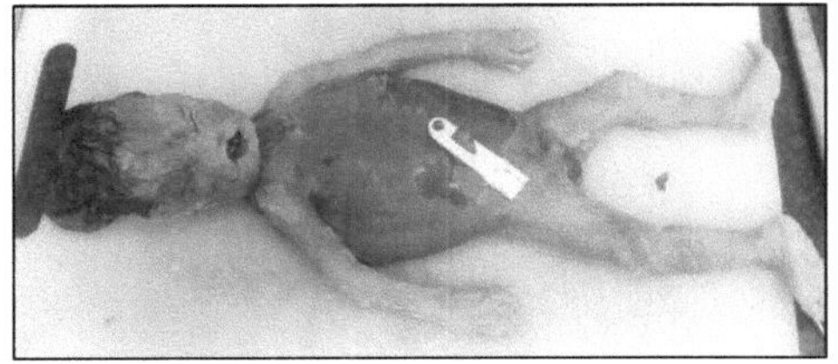

Figure 2: macerated foetus showing epidermolysis (skin detachments), a reddish-brown colour and overlapping skull bones

- The external examination begins with measurements:
- **Weight,**

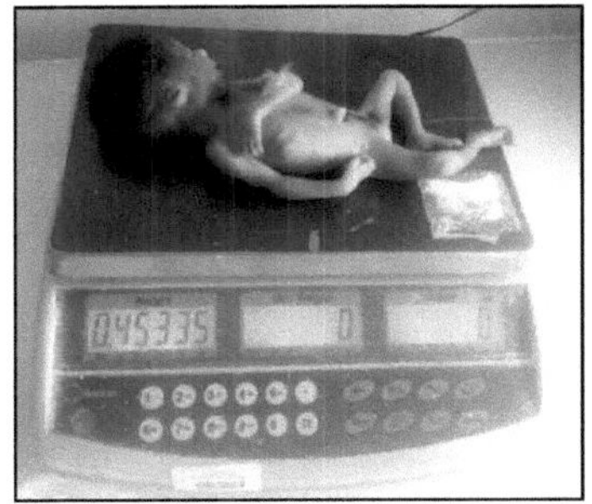

Figure 3: Weighing the foetus.

- **VT** (Vertex- Heel),
- **VC** (Vertex-Coccyx),
- **CP** (Cranial Perimeter),
- **LP** (Foot Length): foot length is used to estimate gestational age using charts (**Fig. 10**).
- **PA** (Abdominal Perimeter): at the level of the umbilicus
- **PT** (Thoracic Perimeter): at the level of the nipples
- **BIP** (Biparietal Diameter),

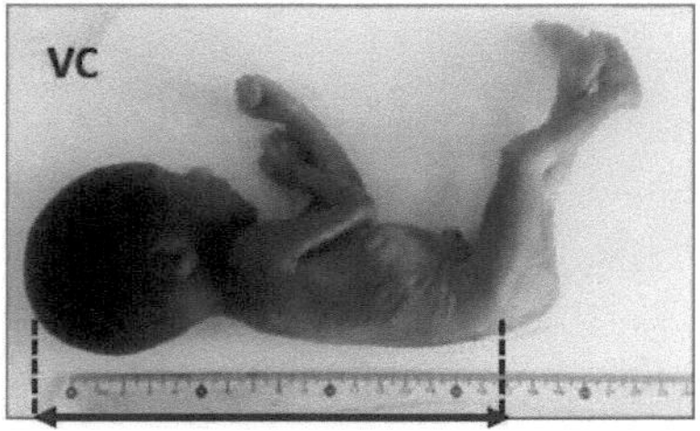

Fig 4: Measuring the Vertex-Coccyx **(VC)** length

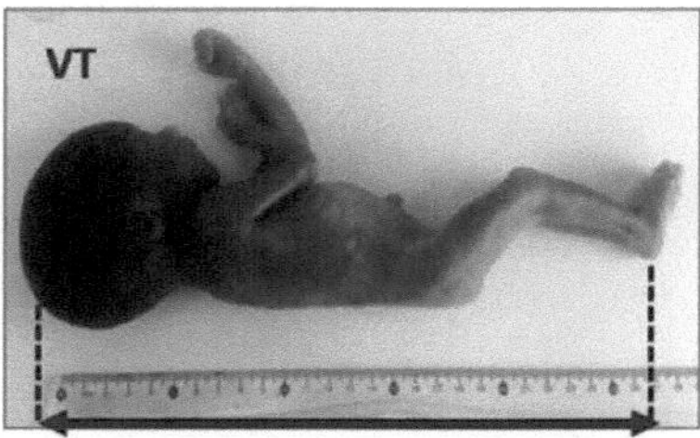

Fig 5: Measuring the Vertex-Talon **(VT)** length

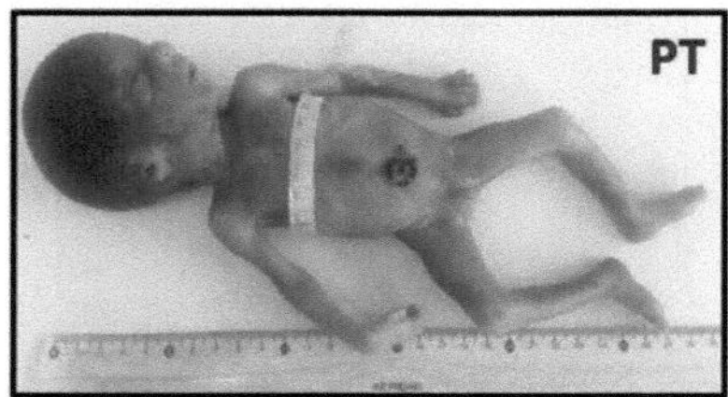

Fig 6: Chest circumference measurement **(TP)**

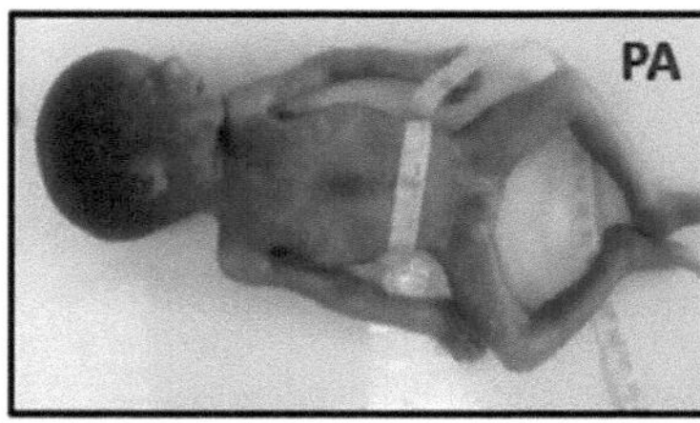

Fig 7: Abdominal circumference measurement **(AP)**

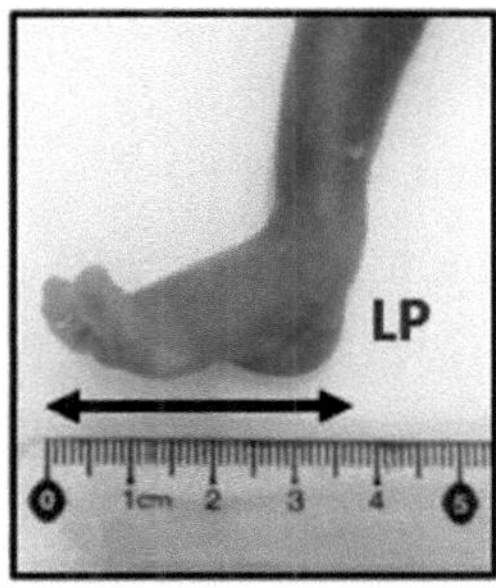

Fig 8: Foot length measurement **(LP)**

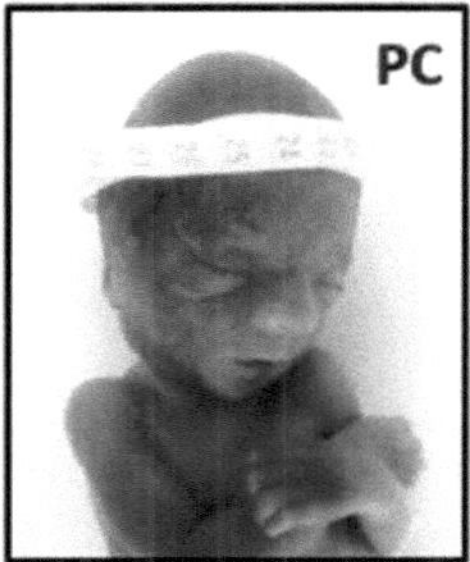

Fig 9: Head circumference measurement **(PC)**

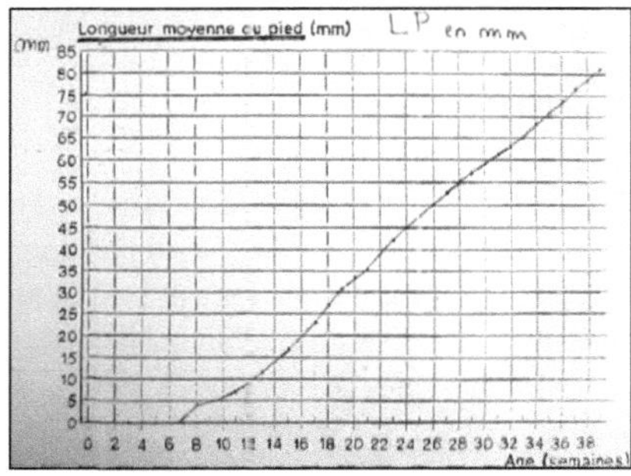

Figure 10: Curve used to estimate gestational age as a function of the foot length.

• **Orifices**: choana, palate, external auditory canal, anus, urethra. The permeability of natural crifices is checked by passing a probe through them: external auditory canal, choanae, anus. We look for a cleft palate and bifid uvula.

- **Cephalic extremity**: fontanelles and sutures, skull bones, face, eyes, mouth, tongue, gums, ears then neck, assessment of facial dysmorphia.

Measurement of inter-canthus distances (Figure 11) :

→ Internal intercanthic distance (DICI) = **CD**

→ External intercanthic distance (DICE) = **AB**

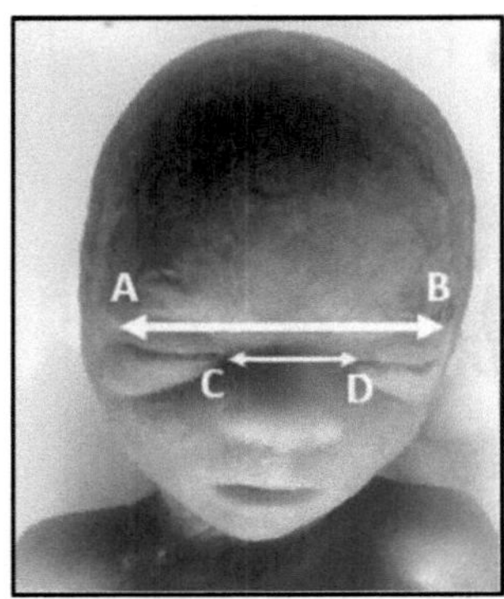

- **Trunk**: anterior face, posterior face, sternum, thorax, abdomen, umbilicus, spine.

- **External genitalia**

- **Limbs**, muscles, extremities and skin.

B. INTERNAL EXAMINATION

After the invertedY incision (Figure 12), the gonads, appendix, gall bladder (to the right of the umbilical vein) and domes are first located, then the sternal plastron is removed. A quick look checks that all the organs are in place, that the heart is on the left, pointing to the left, that the lungs are well lobulated and that there are nositus anomalies. Sterile samples will then be taken for bacteriology and/or virology: lung, liver or DNA from lung, liver, muscle, skin, etc. The samples will be adapted to each case, but the ideal is to systematically keep tissues for DNA for each foetus.

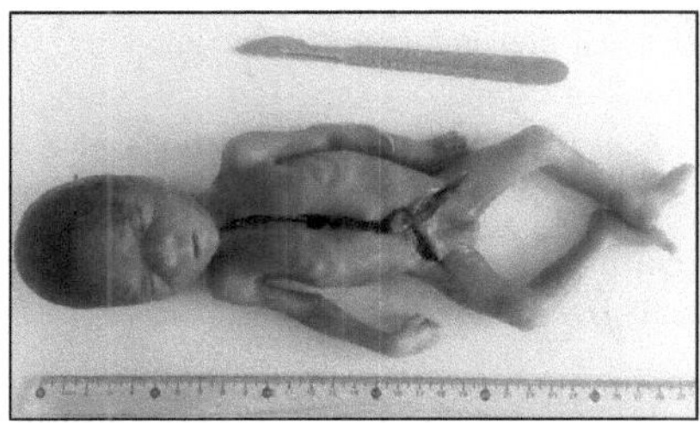

Figure 12: Inverted Y incision for extraction of the visceral monoblock

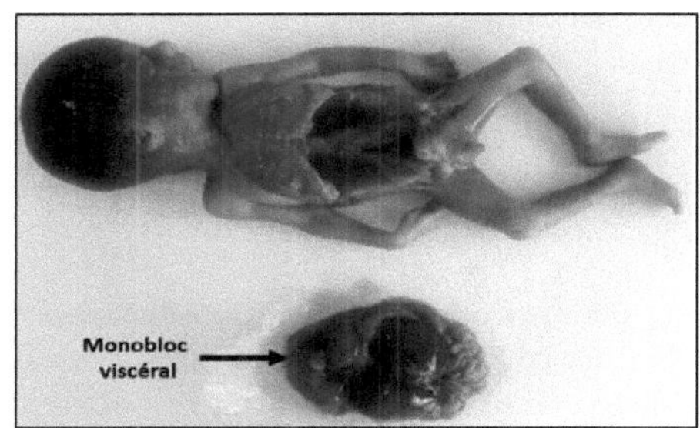

Figure 13: Extraction of the visceral monobloc

The dissection must be meticulous, starting at the top: the **thymus** must be visualised, followed by the **vessels of the neck** and **the heart** with the large vessels, a technique used to examine the heart in situ when the heart is normal. The pulmonary veins must be clearly identified, as abnormal pulmonary venous return may be subdiaphragmatic. If there is heart disease, the heart will be kept in a fixative to be re-examined after being rinsed with formalin by syringe (larsen or formalin). After dissection of the heart, all the vessels in the neck are cut and the heart-lung block is freed by detaching the oesophagus from the spine, checking its patency and that of the trachea and bronchi, and incising the oesophagus to look for an oesotracheal fistula. The aorta can be cut flush with the cupolas and all the viscera weighed and removed for histology. The thyroid gland and larynx can be removed.

The dissection will continue with the abdomino-pelvic stage: removal of the **gonads**, dissection of the **digestive tract** starting at the bottom, then removal from **4 levels** (rectum, colon, small intestine, stomach) dissection of the **pancreas** at the same time, which will be removed with the duodenum at the level of the head of the pancreas, dissection of **the spleen** and **liver**. The **adrenals**, which are moulded onto the **kidneys, and the urinary tract**, which is checked (ureters, bladder and urethra), as well as the renal arteries, remain in place. In the case of megavessia, the kidney-ureters-bladder block is removed and the urethra is opened in the fresh state, which is easier than after fixation in formalin. Lastly, the **internal genital**

organs will be located: **deferens, uterus** in search of an anomaly. **Bone and cartilage** will be taken systematically in cases of chondrodysplasia, ossification anomalies, severe growth retardation, but also in cases of hydrops and viral infections such as **Parvovirus B19** (bone marrow).

Finally, there is the **neuropathological** phase: removal of **the encephalon, which is always** systematic in **cases of foetal pathology**, and is attempted even if the foetus is macerated. Once the brain has been extracted, the usual endocranial structures such as the semicircular canals, etc., are examined. In addition, the **eyes** of all malformed fetuses, particularly those with neurological pathology, and the muscle are removed using conventional histology and electron microscopy. Finally, the **spinal cord** will be systematically sampled in cases of neuromuscular or metabolic pathology.

C. SAMPLES TAKEN FROM THE FOETUS

In addition to the usual sampling of the lung **for bacteriology**, various types of samples may b e taken, for example:

---- **For karyotyping** or **in situ hybridisation**: skin, lung, muscle, ascites, urine and intracardiac blood. Tissues (except blood, which will be sent in a heparinised tube, and urine or ascites in a dry tube) will be immersed in a tube of culture medium kept at 4°C and then placed in a 37°C oven in the Cytogenetics laboratory. These medium tubes can be prepared in advance and kept frozen at -20°, then thawed for use.

→ **For virology**: lung, heart, liver, brain, ascites, intracardiac blood

---- **For cultures for freezing**: skin, lung in many cases of malformative syndromes, metabolic pathology, recurrences, etc.

---- **For electron microscopy**: muscle, skin, other...

---- **For DNA and/or biochemical studies**: muscle, lung, liver, etc. at -80° or in liquid nitrogen for any pathology

In some cases, sampling in isopentane cooled in liquid nitrogen: muscle

CONDITIONS AND RULES OF GOOD PRACTICE

► The foetus must be accompanied by an **information sheet** (Figure 14), which is essential for the examination to be carried out correctly, giving the foetal age, the circumstances of death, family history, the notion of consanguineous union, the progress of the pregnancy, the examinations carried out and their results, ultrasound scans, etc.

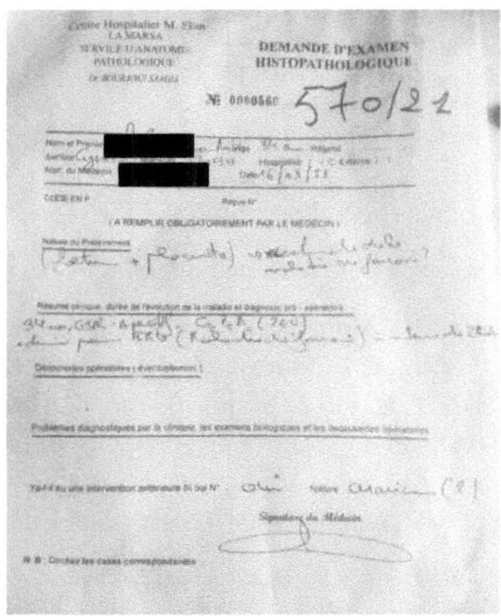

Figure 14: Clinical information sheet

► For an optimal feto-placental examination, the fetus and placenta must arrive at the pathology laboratory in a fresh state as soon as possible after expulsion. They must not have been frozen.

► Fixation makes it impossible to take special samples: to test for infection, freeze for DNA extraction or histo-enzymological analysis.

► All the parameters will be recorded on a written document, including the weight and measurements of the foetus. All abnormalities will be noted, whether during the external or internal examination.

CONCLUSION

■ The foetopathological examination is the same for all foetuses; additional examinations or samples must be adapted to each case. This examination must be optimal in order to provide parents with the most accurate genetic advice.

■ The foetopathology report must be clear and concise, highlighting any anomalies and not getting bogged down in unnecessary detail. It is important to bear in mind that this report can be read by the parents, so no zoological comparisons (batrachian facies) and above all that this document, together with the photos, X-rays and results of the foetopathological examination, must be clear and concise. of all the tests should enable parents to be given informed genetic advice.

REFERENCES

1) Fetal autopsy: a relevant medical procedure | Documents de Médecine Légale (wordpress.com)

2) Kalousek DK. Pathology of abortion: the embryo and the previable fetus. In Gilbert-

Barness E (ed.). Potter's pathology of the fetus and infant. St. Louis: Mosby; 1997. p. 106.

3) Emmrich P, Horn LC, Seifert U. [Morphologic findings in fetuses and placentas of late abortion in the 2nd trimester]. Zentralbl Gynakol. 1998;120(8):399-405.

4) Marton T, Hargitai B, Patkós P, Csapó Z, Szende B, Papp Z. [Practice of fetal pathological examination]. [Practice of fetal pathological examination. Orv Hetil. 1999 Jun 20;140(25):1411-6.

5) Pathologic Examination of Fetal and Placental Tissue Obtained by Dilation and Evacuation

| Archives of Pathology & Laboratory Medicine | Allen Press

TECHNICAL SHEET: MACROSCOPIC MANAGEMENT OF A MYOMECTOMY SPECIMEN

GENERAL

▪ Uterine myoma, also known as leiomyoma, is a mesenchymal tumour that develops in the smooth muscle, often separated from the myometrium by a pseudo-capsule linked to the condensation of connective tissue.

▪ It is a benign hormone-dependent tumour, increasing in size during pregnancy and under estrogen treatment, and regressing at the menopause.

METHODOLOGY

A- Reports

The position of the largest transverse diameter of the myomas in relation to the myometrium will enable them to be classified into three families:

• **Submucosal myomas**: lifting up the endometrium and bulging into the uterine cavity

• **Intramural or interstitial myomas**: in the myometrial wall

• **Subserosal myomas**: raise the serosa and bulge into the peritoneal cavity

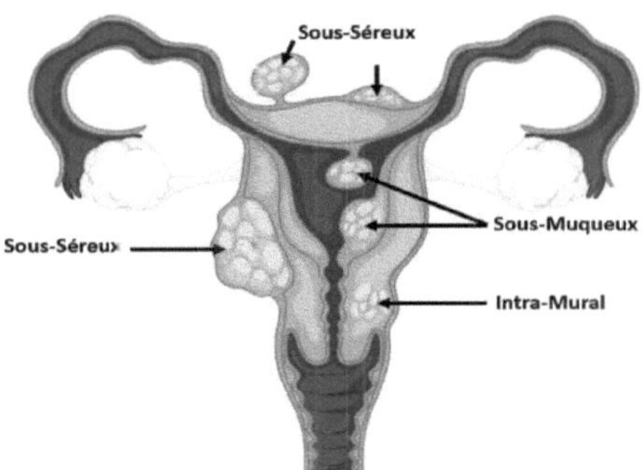

Figure 1: Location of leiomyomas
Uterine Fibroids - Gynaecology and Obstetrics - MSD Manual Professional Edition
(msdmanuals.com)

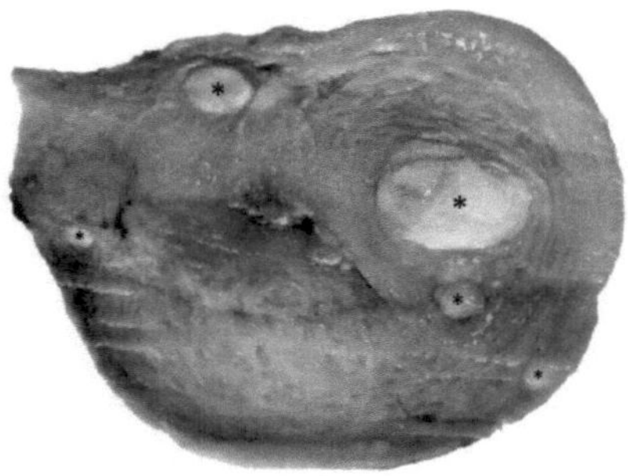

Figure 2: Intramural leiomyomas on a hysterectomy specimen (asterisks)

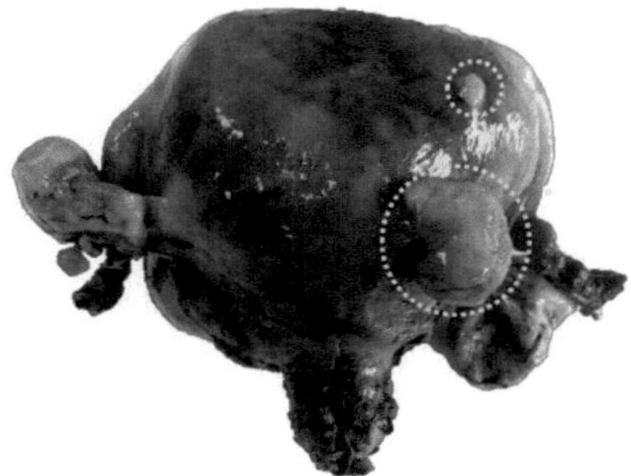

Figure 3: Two subserosal leiomyomas on a hysterectomy specimen

B- Referral criteria

No referral possible for myomectomy where leiomyomas are often transmitted separately

C- Weigh all uterine leiomyomas

- Overall Igrams

- Possibly individually for larger items

D- Describe uterine leiomyomas

- Number of leiomyomas
- Size of leiomyomas, from largest to smallest
- the three dimensions of the largest
- the largest dimension of the smallest

E- Opening leiomyomas

Open them all and specify :
- The **colour**

- The presence of areas of necrosis	□ yes	□ no
- Haemorrhagic changes	□ yes	□ no
- Edematous changes	□ yes	□ no
- Calcifications	□ yes	□ no
F- Sampling In the absence of a reshuffle		

Systematically remove **1 block** for each large leiomyoma (**>5cm**)

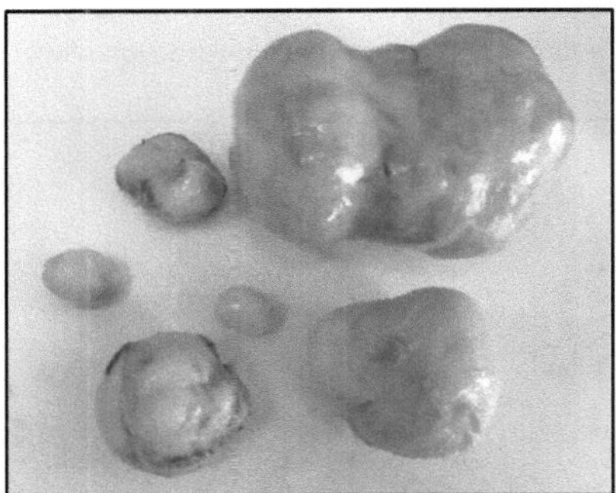

Figure 4: Macroscopic appearance of numerous uterine leiomyomas

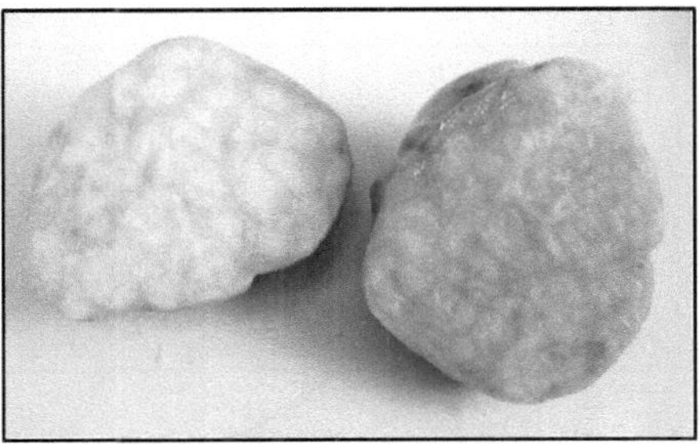

Figure 5: Macroscopic appearance of a non-remodeled uterine leiomyoma: On section: homogeneous fasciculated whitish.

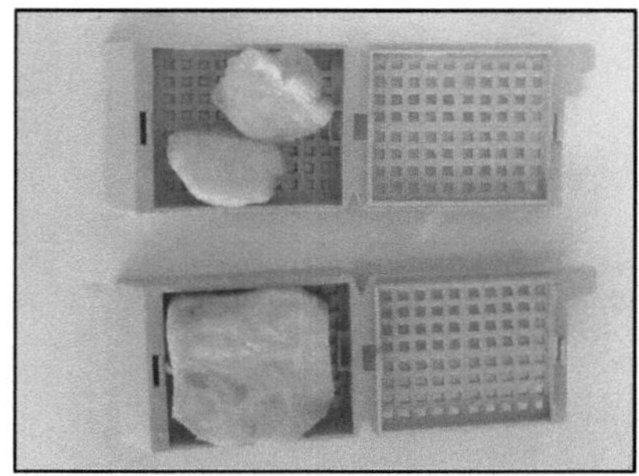

Figure 6: Samples taken from myomas are placed in cassettes

- **In the event of reshuffles**

☐ Always remove **1 block per cm of longest axis,** whatever the size of the myoma.

☐ In the event of fragmentation due to the surgical technique, measurement is not possible and a slice should be systematically taken from each resection chip.

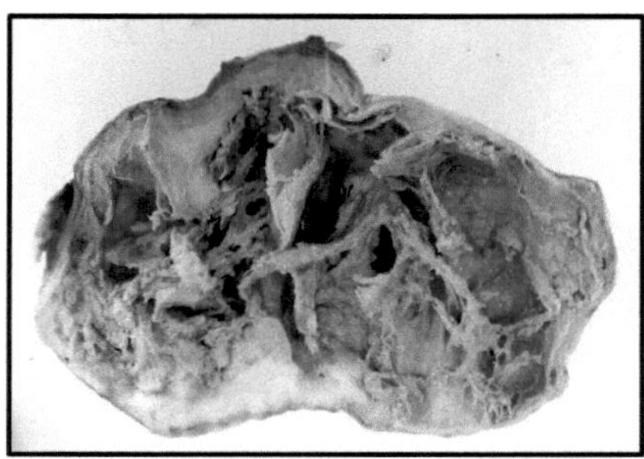

Figure 7: Remanufactured leiomyoma in aseptic necrobiosis with cystic degeneration

MATERIAL REQUIRED

11. Fixing agent: The usual fixing agent is 10% buffered formalin.

12. Scalpel blade - knife

13. Scissors

14. Tape measure - Flat ruler

15. Cassettes

16. Camera

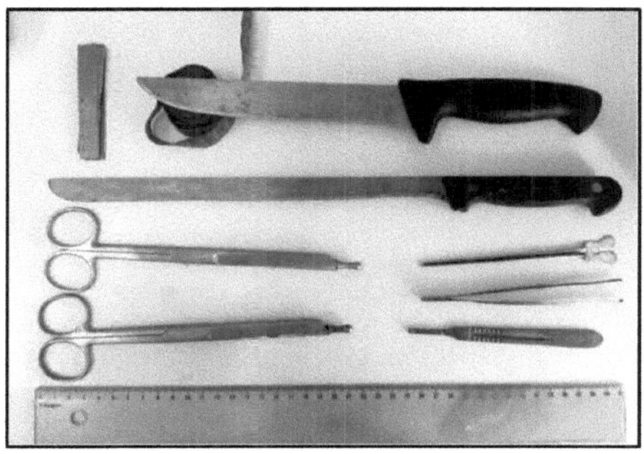

Figure 8: Equipment required for macroscopic processing of Myomectomy Parts

CONDITIONS AND RULES OF GOOD PRACTICE

- The surgical specimen is fixed for 24 - 48 hours in 10% buffered formalin.
- Delayed or poor fixation will affect the morphological quality of histological sections. Respect the ratio of tissue volume to fixative volume (1/10).
- All myomectomy specimens must be sent to the pathological anatomy laboratory together with a clinical information sheet describing the history of the disease, the patient's background, the results of the paraclinical examinations carried out and the treatment administered.

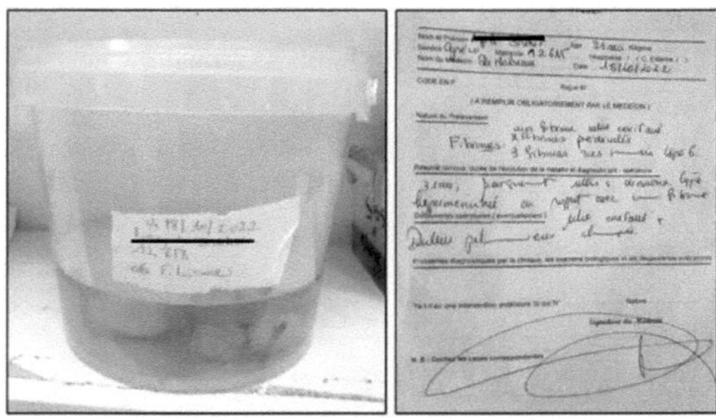

Figure 9: Six formalin-fixed myomectomy specimens in a labelled vial, accompanied by a clinical information sheet.

CONCLUSION

- Macroscopic examination of myomectomy specimens contributes to patient management.
- He must be methodical and meticulous.
- Adequate sampling must be carried out on the myomectomy specimens in order to to eliminate malignancy.

REFERENCES

1. 9 Item.pdf (lsmuni.lt)
2. course.pdf (confkhalifa.com)

TECHNICAL SHEET: MACROSCOPIC MANAGEMENT OF A SIMPLE ADNEXECTOMY SPECIMEN

ANATOMICAL REMINDER
Ovary

- Its volume varies according to the period of genital activity and atrophies after the menopause.
- Its surface is irregularly bumpy during the period of genital activity, in related to the maturation and rupture of follicles.

Reports from the ovary

- The **ovarian hilum** is attached to the back of the broad ligament by the **meso-ovarium**.
- The utero-ovarian ligament attaches the medial border of the ovary to the uterine horn. below and behind the proboscis.
- The lumbo-ovarian ligament (or infundibulo-pelvic ligament) attaches the upper pole of the ovary to the pelvic wall and participates in vascularisation via the lumbo-ovarian vessels (collateral of the aorta and the IVC).

Uterine tube

The horn has **4 parts**:

- **The infundibulum (pinna)**, distal portion, 10 mm long.
- **The ampulla** is half the length of the tube, narrower and more tortuous.
- **The isthmus** is 20 to 30 mm long with a narrow lumen and a thick, more muscular wall.
- And **the interstitial** (or intramural) **portion**, where the muscularis joined the myometrium.
- **Size**: 9 to 12 cm long, but after fixing it often appears shorter and more compact.

sinuous due to the size of the muscularis.

Relationships of the uterine tube

- The proximal limit of the tube is attached to the uterine horn above and in front of the ovarian ligament and above and behind the round ligament of the uterus.

- The pelvic peritoneum reflects on the tube to give the **meso-salpinx**, on the ovarian ligament to give the **meso-ovarium** and on the round ligament to give the broad ligament.

METHODOLOGY
Referral criteria
- Specify **laterality**:
- □ **Right**
- □ **Left**
- The tube is covered by a fold of peritoneum forming the **meso-salpinx**.
- The ovarian vessels are covered by a fold of peritoneum **known as the meso-ovarium**.
- The uterine tube and meso-salpinx are **in front of** the ovary and meso-ovarium.
- At the level of the uterine horn, the insertion of the uterine horn, the uterine tube and the vessels of the ovary, which continue into the parametrium, can be seen from front to back.

Separating the ovary and managing it

Separating the ovary from the fallopian tube
Measuring the ovary :
Weigh the ovary alone:
Open the ovary in a cutting plane passing through the ovarian hilum

Describe any ovarian lesions:

- □ Cysts
- □ Yellow body
- □ Fibrous remodelling
- □ Haemorrhagic changes.

(Remove these lesions)

Systematically remove a slice of ovarian section passing through the hilum: **1 block**
Management of the uterine tube

Measuring the uterine tube :

Length:
Describe any tubal lesions:

- **Paratubal cyst**
- **Tubal dilatation**
- **Tube clips**
- **Salpingotomy**

▪ Haematoma of the wall .

Removing these lesions

Systematically take three staggered cross-sectional slices from 1 block

▪ 1 proximal isthmic slice

▪ 1 medium ampullary slice

▪ 1 pavilion distal slice

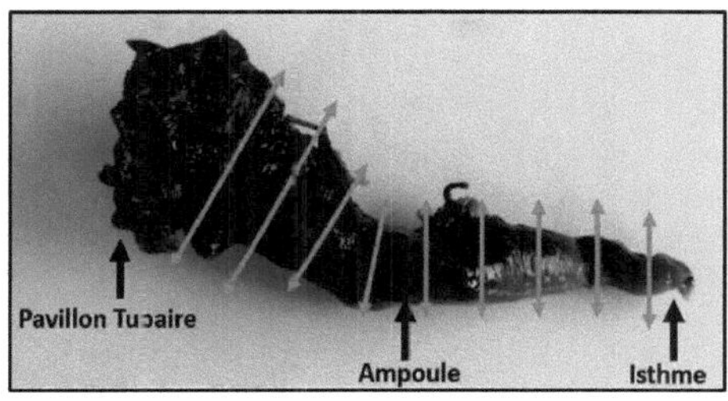

Figure 1: Samples taken from the tube after serial slicing

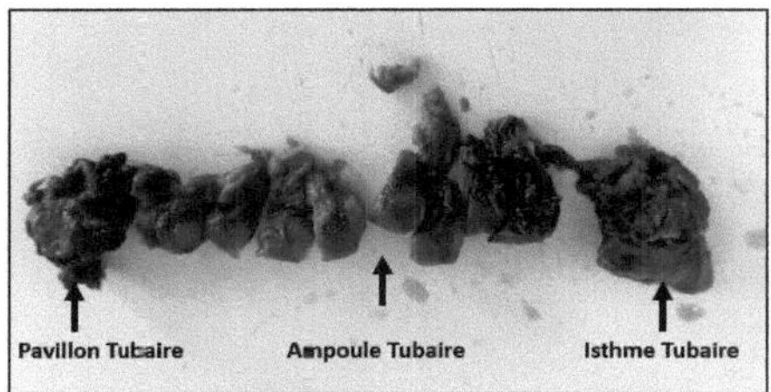

Figure 2: Samples taken from the tube after serial slicing

What to sample
OVAIRE
1 section slice passing through the hilum of the ovary□ 1 block
UTERINE TRUMP
3 tubular stepped transverse slices□ 1 block Remove any associated lesion(s)

MATERIAL REQUIRED

17. Fixing agent: The usual fixing agent is 10% buffered formalin.

18. Scalpel blade - knife

19. Scissors

20. **Tape measure - Flat ruler**

21. **Cassettes**

22. **Camera**

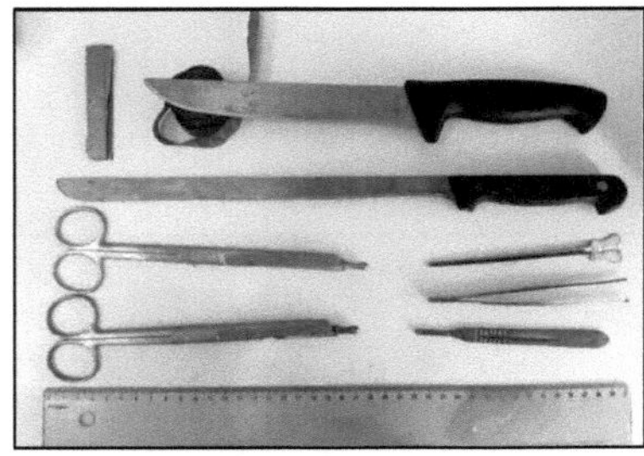

Figure 3: Equipment required for macroscopic management of intestinal resection specimens

EXAMPLES OF ADNEXECTOMY PARTS

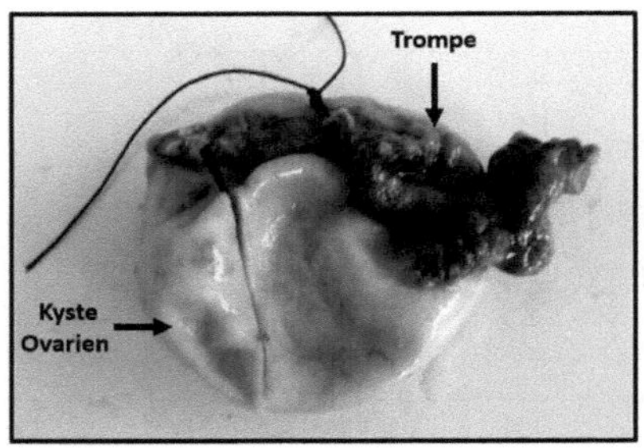

Figure 4: Adnexectomy specimen with a tube and ovary containing a unilocular serous cyst.

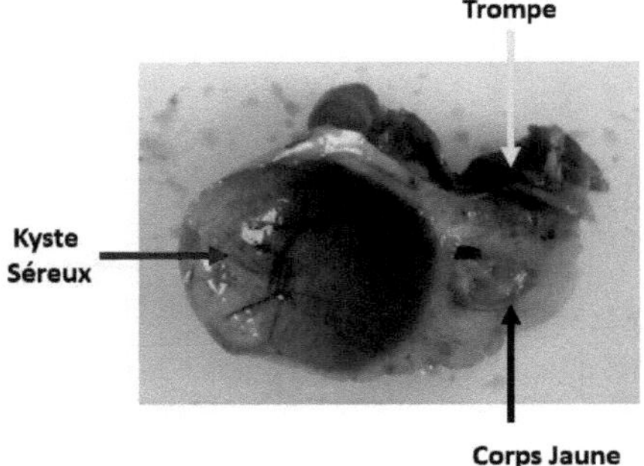

Figure 5: Adnexectomy specimen with a tube and ovary containing a unilocular serous cyst and corpus luteum.

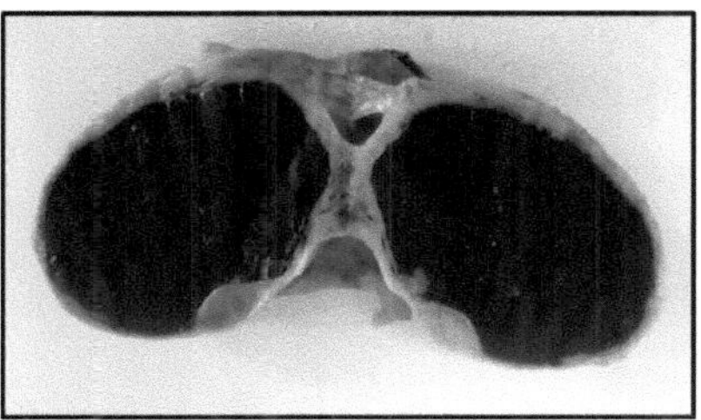

Figure 6: Adnexectomy specimen with an ovary containing a unilocular endometriotic cyst with "chocolate" haemorrhagic content.

CONDITIONS AND RULES OF GOOD PRACTICE

- The surgical specimen is fixed for 24 - 48 hours in 10% buffered formalin.
- Delayed or poor fixation will affect the morphological quality of the histological sections. Respect the ratio of tissue volume to fixative volume (1/10).
- All adnexectomy specimens must be sent to the pathological anatomy laboratory together with a clinical information sheet describing the history of the disease, the patient's history, the results of the paraclinical examinations carried out and the treatment administered.

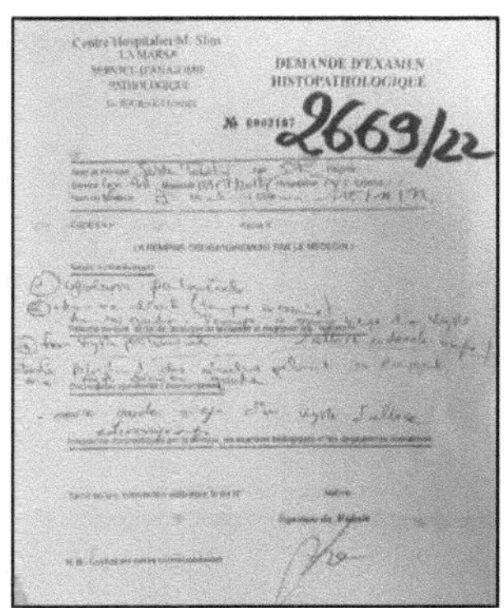

Figure 7: Clinical information sheet accompanying a part adnexectomy report received by the pathology laboratory

CONCLUSION

- Macroscopic examination of adnexectomy specimens contributes to patient management by assessing prognosis and defining important criteria for prescribing any additional postoperative treatment.

REFERENCES
3. The-Ovaries.pdf (uca.ma)
4. Les-Trompes-utérines.pdf (uca.ma)
5. UTERINE TRUMPS (univ-batna2.dz)
6. Layout 1 (cngof.net)

TECHNICAL SHEET: MACROSCOPIC MANAGEMENT OF AN OVARIAN CYSTECTOMY SPECIMEN

GENERAL

An ovarian cyst is a fluid-containing swelling that develops at the expense of the ovaries. Ovarian cysts are subdivided into functional cysts and organic cysts.
- **Functional cysts** are the most common. They occur in women during periods of genital activity. Functional cysts are due to a "hormonal imbalance" which causes a follicle or physiological corpus luteum to transform into a cyst.
- **Organic cysts** develop at the expense of the surface epithelium (epithelial tumours of the ovary), specialised stroma (sexual cord tumours) or germ cells (germ cell tumours of the ovary). These tumours are usually benign, but may be of limited malignancy (borderline tumour of the ovary) or malignant.

METHODOLOGY

A- Measure and weigh the cyst

■ **Cyst communicated :**

□ **Intact**
□ **Open**

■ **Measuring** the cyst
■ Or in its two dimensions, if open

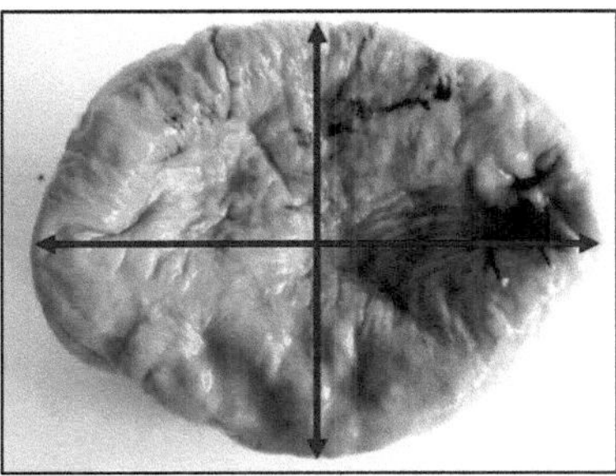

Figure 1: Measurement of a serous cystadenoma that has been opened in its two main dimensions

Weigh the cyst
If it has arrived intact (unopened) and is of significant size (> 5cm)

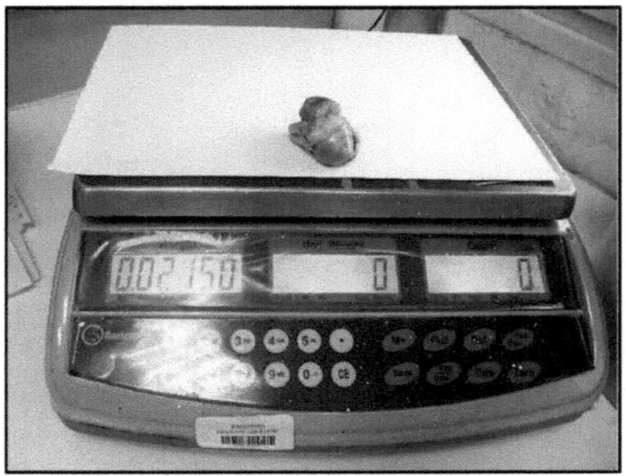

Figure 2: Weighing the cyst

B- Describe the external surface of the cyst

Watch the clip :

□ **Capsule intact**
□ **Suspicion of capsular rupture**

Its outer walls :

□ **Smooth walls**
□ **External vegetation**

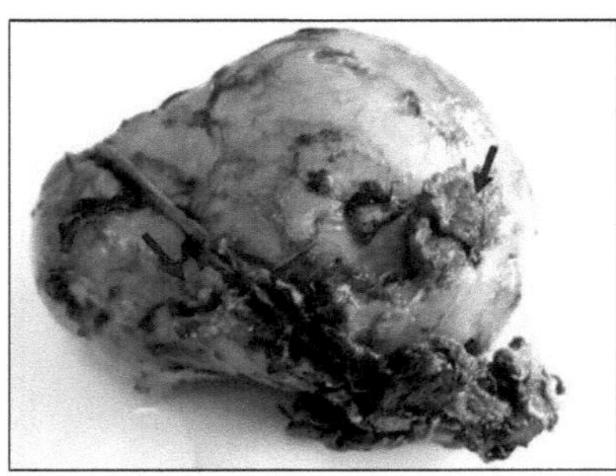

Figure 3: External surface of an ovarian cyst with exocystic vegetations(blue arrows)

If vegetation or capsular rupture is suspected: **ink the external surface**

C- Open the cyst and describe its contents

Open the cyst (beware of splashing)

Describe its contents

□ **Serous**

□ **Mucinous**

□ **Hemorrhagic/chocolate**

□ **Cloudy**

□ **Hair residue**

□ **Other :**

D- Describe the inner surface of the cyst

Type
□ **Unilocular**
□ **Multilocular**

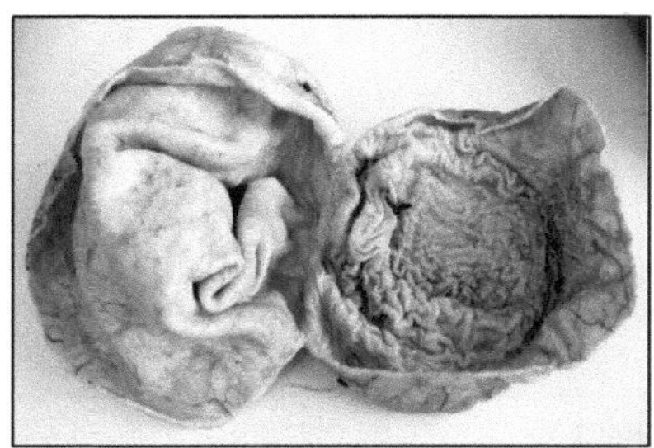

Figure 4 : Unilocular cystic formation (Serous cystadenoma)

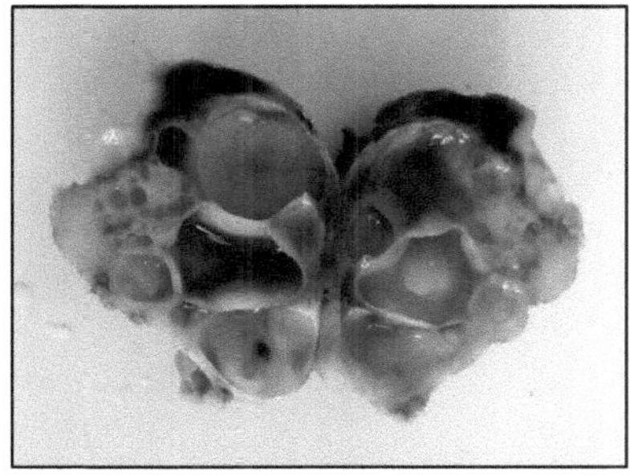

Figure 5: Multilocular cystic formation (Mucinous cystadenoma)

Describe its internal walls :
Smooth wallsInternal vegetation
Presence of any solid areas and their proportion
Solid (%)

E- Sampling the ovarian tumour
□ **Serous fluid cyst**
cyst < 5 cm with a smooth-walled serous fluid appearance: Remove 1 block
cyst > 5cm, serous fluid with a smooth wall:
Take 2 to 3 blocks
□ **Mucinous fluid cyst**
cyst < 3 cm with mucinous fluid appearance: Include all
cyst > 3 cm with mucinous fluid appearance: Include 1 block/cm
□ **Haemorrhagic cyst / chocolate**
cyst of any size: Include 1 block/cm

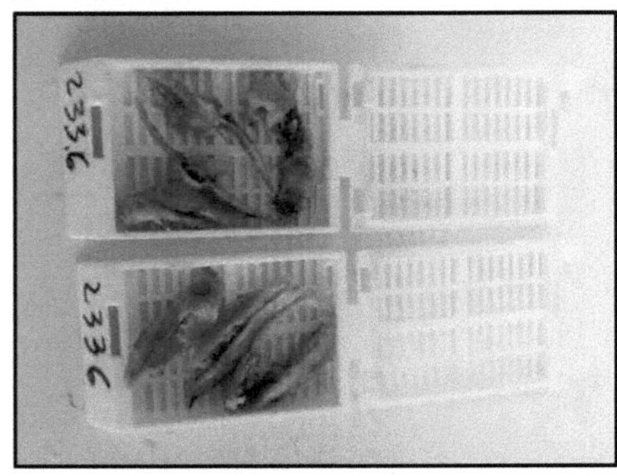

Figure 6: samples taken from an ovarian cyst are placed in cassettes

▪ **Cyst with vegetations all vegetations** must be removed, up to **a** maximum of **one block per cm,** whatever the size of the cyst.

▪ **Cyst with solid component** solid territories must be removed **at a** rate of **one block per cm.**

MATERIAL REQUIRED
23. Fixing agent: The usual fixing agent is 10% buffered formalin.
24. Scalpel blade - knife
25. Scissors
26. Tape measure - Flat ruler
27. Cassettes
28. Camera

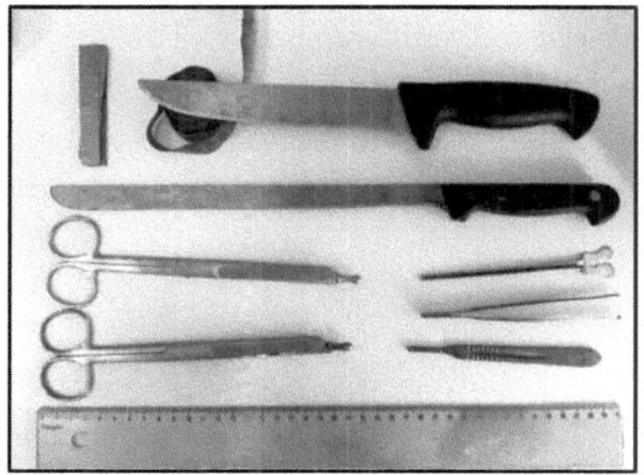

Figure 7: Equipment required for macroscopic management of intestinal resection specimens

I. EXAMPLES OF OVARIAN CYSTECTOMY SPECIMENS

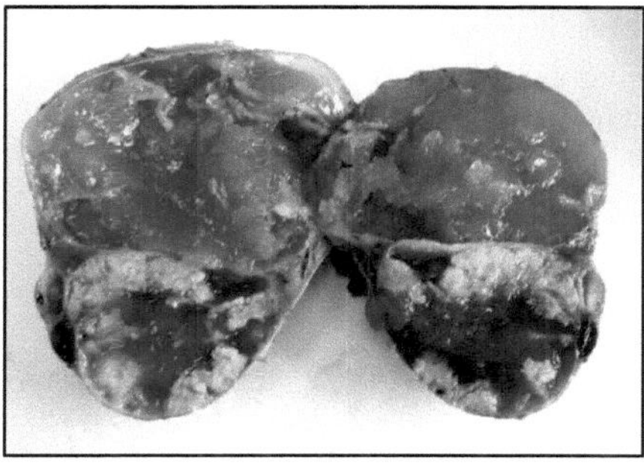

Figure 8: Bilocular ovarian cystic formation with gelatinous, viscous content and solid component

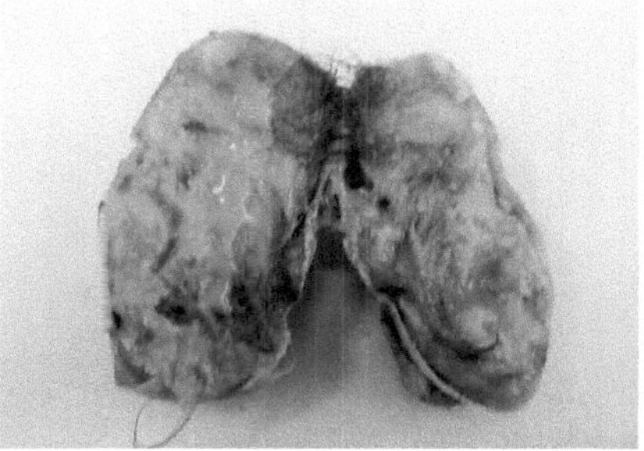

Figure 9 : Unilocular cystic formation with pilosebaceous content (mature cystic teratoma)

CONDITIONS AND RULES OF GOOD PRACTICE

- The surgical specimen is fixed for 24 - 48 hours in 10% buffered formalin.
- Delayed or poor fixation will affect the morphological quality of the histological sections.

31

Respect the ratio of tissue volume to fixative volume (1/10).

▪ All ovarian cystectomy specimens must be sent to the pathological anatomy laboratory together with a clinical information sheet describing the history of the disease, the patient's history, the results of the paraclinical examinations carried out and the treatment administered.

CONCLUSION

▪ Macroscopic examination of ovarian cystectomy specimens contributes to patient management by specifying the histological type of cyst and assessing prognosis.

REFERENCES

7. Ovarian cysts.pdf (miniseminaires.com)

8. Microsoft Word - Ovarian cyst.docx_3rd_year [1] (facmed-univ- oran.dz)

9. Item-153-Lovary-smoking-course.pdf (confkhalifa.com)

TECHNICAL SHEET: MACROSCOPIC EXAMINATION OF A HYSTERECTOMY SPECIMEN

ANATOMICAL REMINDER

- The uterus is an odd, median organ located in the pelvic cavity.
- It is shaped like a truncated cone, with an upper base and a lower apex.
- It has a constriction in the middle: this is the uterine isthmus, which divides the organ into two parts:
- One above the uterine body.
- the lower one the cervix
- The uterine wall is made up of 3 layers, from surface to depth:

1. **Peritoneal serosa** or **perimeter**: exists only in the body.
The isthmus and cervix have no peritoneum.

2. **The muscularis** or **myometrium**: very thick, it is made up of 3 layers:
external, middle and internal. It is an involuntary smooth muscle.

3. **The mucous membrane**: thin and friable, it forms the endometrium in the body.

- The uterus has 3 segments:
- Body
- Isthmus
- Collar
- **Body:** Triangular in shape. It features :
- Two sides
- Three angles
- Three edges

Several regions can be isolated:
- The right and left uterine horns
- The uterine fundus
- Anterior surface: curved opposite the recto-vesical pouch
- The posterior surface opposite the cul de sac of Douglas (recto-uterine cul de sac).

- **The isthmus :**
The isthmus is a virtual region at the junction between the uterine body and the cervix.
- Its non-peritonealised outer surface is at the junction between the parametrium and the paracervix.
- Its wall lies between the fibro-muscular wall of the cervix and the myometrium of the body.
- Its mucosa lies at the junction between the endocervix and the endometrium.

■ **Peritoneum** :

The upper part of the uterus is covered by the peritoneal serosa, which is reflected :

- Forward to form the vesico-uterine cul-de-sac

- Backwards to form the recto-uterine cul-de-sac (cul-de-sac of Douglas)

The peritoneum reflects on the adnexa to form :

- **Meso-salpinx** on the fallopian tubes

- **Meso-ovarii** on ovarian vessels

Parameters and paracervix :

The peritoneum reflects to form :

- The **mesosalpinx** on the fallopian tubes

- **Meso-ovarii** on ovarian vessels

- The parametrium are arranged laterally to the uterine body and include vessels and the right and left parametrial ligaments.

- The **paracervixes**: are arranged laterally to the cervix and contain vessels and the right and left paracervical ligaments.

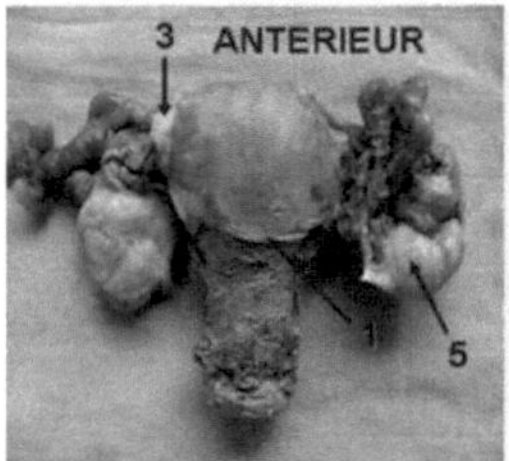
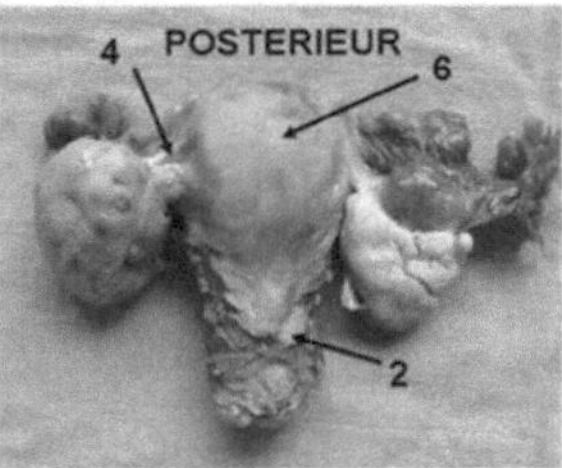

Figure 1: **1.** vesico-uterine cul-de-sac (higher); **2.** recto-uterine cul-de-sac (Douglas); **3.** round ligament; **4.** Utero-ovarian ligament; **5.** Posterior surface of uterus (more rounded)

DEFINITIONS :

⬇ **Appendix**: ovary + uterine tube

⬇ **Subtotal hysterectomy**: Leaves the cervix in place

⬇ **Total hysterectomy**: removal of the cervix

⬇ **Inter-annexal or conservative hysterectomy**: leaves the adnexa in place

⬇ **Extended colpo-hysterectomy**: uterus (body and neck) + parametrium / paracervix + vaginal collar

⬇ **Trachelectomy**: removal of the cervix and paracervix with vaginal collar that can be extended to the parameters

⬇ **Colpectomy**: removal of a vaginal fragment

⬇ **Anterior pelvectomy**: bladder + uterus + vagina

34

⬦ Posterior **pelvectomy**: uterus + vagina + rectum
⬦ **Total pelvectomy**: bladder + uterus + vagina + rectum

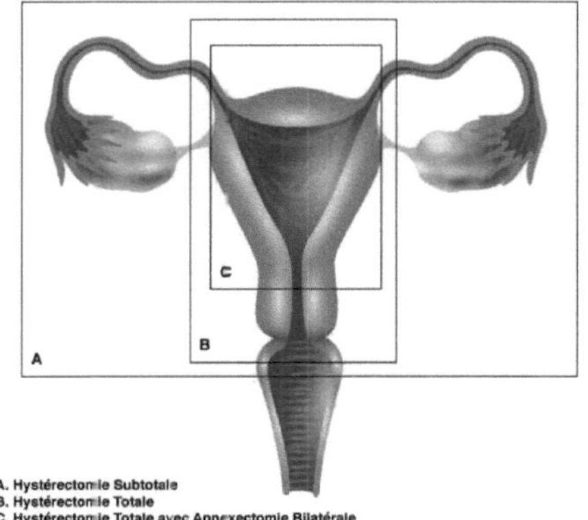

Figure 2: Types of intervention
Hysterectomy - surgical and robotic expertise (gynecomarseille.com)

METHODOLOGY

1. Orientation of the operating room :

Guidance criteria :

■ **Curved posterior** surface of uterus
■ Serosa of the cul de sac of Douglas (posterior) descends **lower** than the serosa of the vesico-uterine cul de sac
■ Uterine horns from front to back :
- round ligament
- mesosalpinx
- meso-ovarium
■ Trompes in front of the ovaries

2. Appendices

Differentiating and separating the Right and Left annexes
Block **tubes** (right and left tubes)
■ **Straight horn :**
■ Length: ‖ mm

Diameter: ׀ mm

■ **Trompe gauche :** Length: ׀ mm

Diameter: ׀ mm
If there is no macroscopic lesion, at least 1 block per tube with 3 levels (isthmus / ampulla / infundibulum), isolating the right and left.

Ovarian blocks (right and left ovaries)
■ **Measure** ovaries: ׀׀ ׀ x ׀׀ ׀ mm
■ **Weighing** the ovaries: ׀   ׀׀grams

If there is no macroscopic lesion, at least 1 block per ovary, isolating the right ovary from the left.In the case of macroscopic lesions, please refer to the macroscopic management of adnexa.

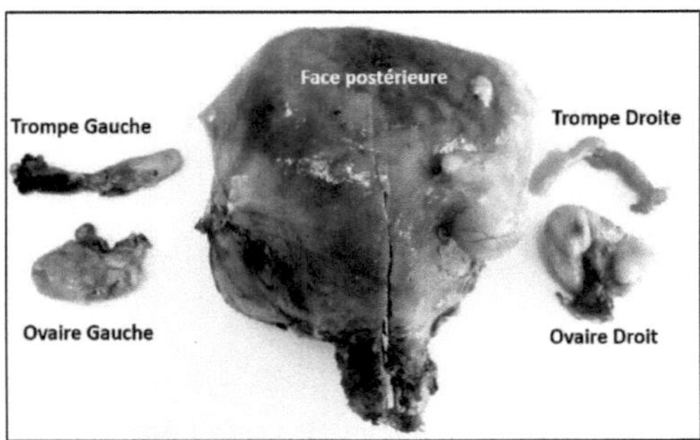

Figure 3: Differentiation and separation of the Right and Left appendices

3. Weighing the uterus
■ **Weigh**

The uterus: ׀׀ ׀ grams

■ **No inking** in the absence of tumour pathology

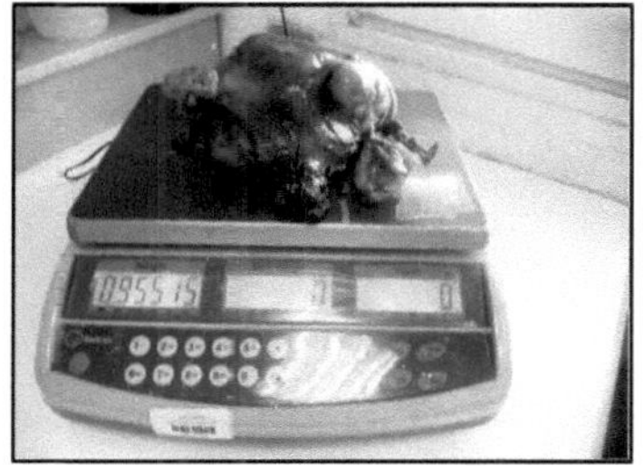

Figure 4: weighing the hysterectomy specimen

4. Isthmus

■ Cross-section of the isthmus

■ Make an incision on the left side (for example)

5. Uterine cervix

■ Measure collar: → Height ǀ ǁ mm
→ Diameter ǁ mm

■ **Catheterise** with a fine cannula
■ **Cut into serial vertical slices** blocks C1 to C...
■ No macroscopic lesion: take at least two sagittal slices, including the anterior and posterior lips.

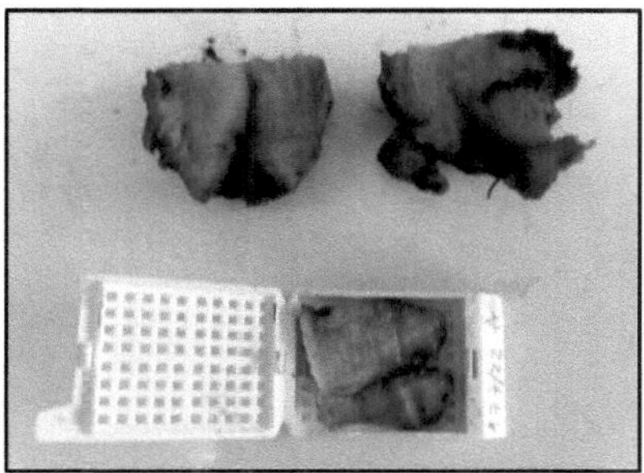

Figure 5: Cervical sampling

■ **Non-malignant lesions** (e.g. uterine leiomyomas) :
---- Describe and locate them
---- Collecting them

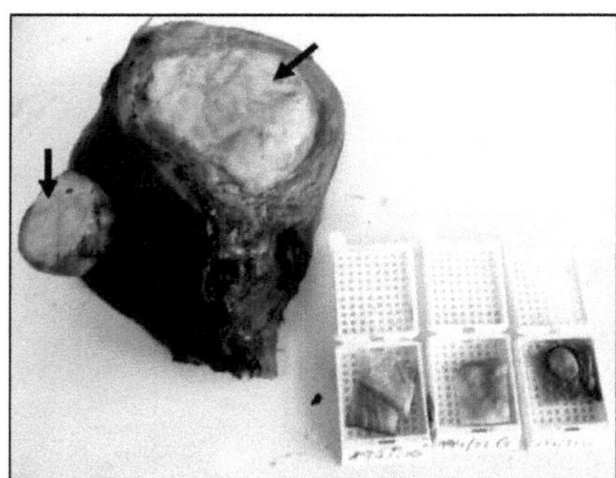

Figure 6: Sampling and description of uterine leiomyomas (black arrows) on a total hysterectomy specimen.

6. Harvesting uterine horns:

Optional

Remove the uterine horns from a block, isolating the right and left horns.

7. Uterine body :

■ **Measuring** the uterine body :
■ **Catheterising** the uterine lumen
■ **Cut in serial vertical slices** along the cannula, isolating the right and left sections.

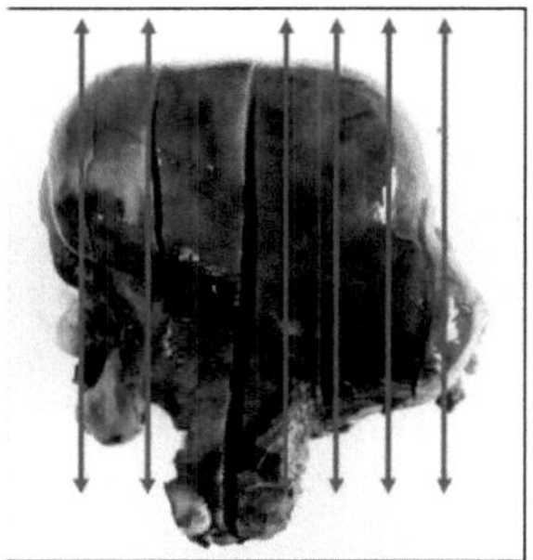

Figure 7: Serial vertical slices of the uterine body

■ **Describe the endometrium**
- Endometrial thickness |ı | mm
- Describe any lesions, locate and remove them

■ **Describe the myometrium**

- Myometrial thickness |ı | mm
- Remodelling of the wall o yes o no
- Uterine myomas: number|

Size of largest |ı | mm

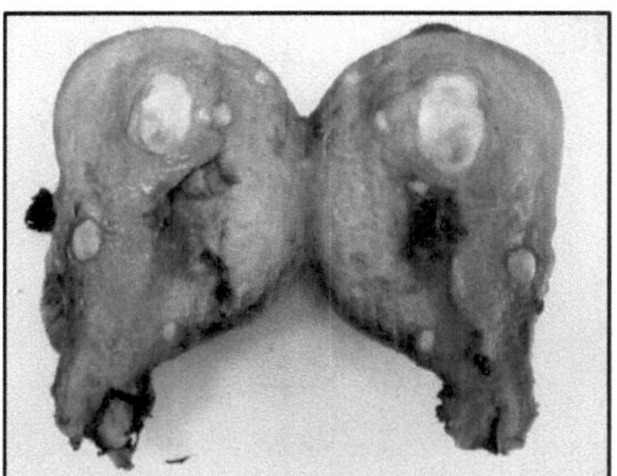

Figure 8: Total hysterectomy specimen showing a large number of intramural leiomyomas on section.

■ Sample **a complete sagittal midline slice** to be included in its **entirety**, specifying the topography of blocks E1 to E...

Summary: What to sample

- **Appendices :**
If no lesion: 1 block per uterine tube and per ovary
- **Isthmus :**
- **Collar:**
At least 2 blocks on a sagittal slice allowing examination of the anterior and posterior lips
(12 hours and 6 hours)
- **Uterine body :**
A complete sagittal slice :
At least two blocks at best 4 blocks
Remove any endo-uterine lesions, polyps or myomas
- **Uterine horns:** 1 slice per uterine horn (optional)

MATERIAL REQUIRED

1. **Fixing agent:** The usual fixing agent is 10% buffered formalin.
2. **Scalpel blade - knife**
3. **Scissors**
4. **Tape measure - Flat ruler**
5. **Cassettes**
6. **Camera**

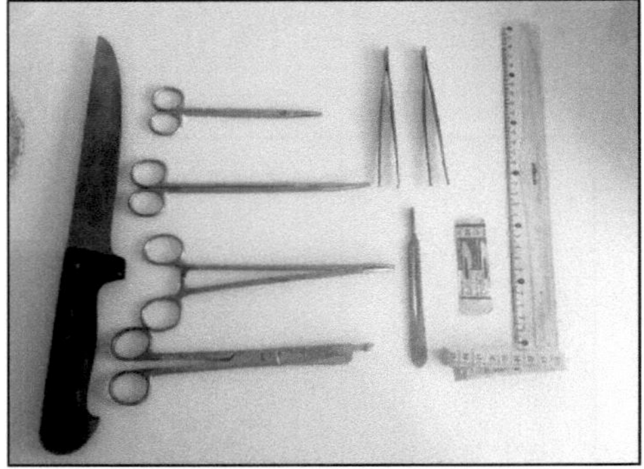

Figure 9: Equipment required for macroscopic management of cephalic duodeno-pancreatectomy specimens
(Photo of the pathological anatomy department of the CHU Mongi Slim La Marsa)

CONDITIONS AND RULES OF GOOD PRACTICE

▪ The surgical specimen is fixed for 24 - 48 hours in 10% buffered formalin.
▪ Delayed or poor fixation will affect the morphological quality of histological sections.
Respect the ratio of tissue volume to fixative volume (1/10).
▪ All hysterectomy specimens must be sent to the pathological anatomy laboratory together
with a clinical information sheet describing the history of the disease, the patient's
background, the results of the paraclinical examinations carried out and the treatment
administered.

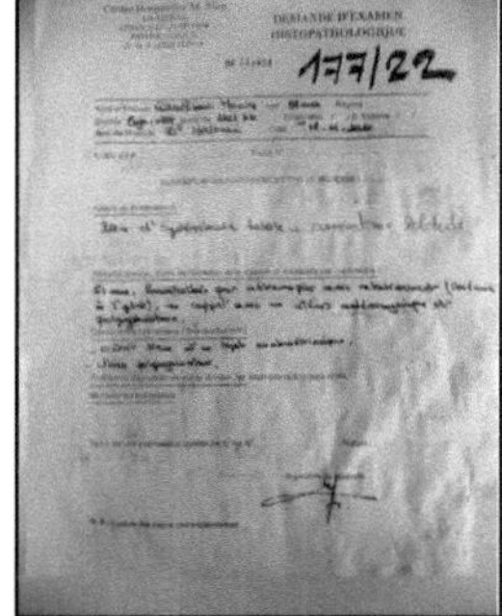

Figure 10: Pathology request form

CONCLUSION

▪ Macroscopic examination of hysterectomy specimens contributes to patient management
by assessing prognosis and defining important criteria for prescribing any additional
postoperative treatment.

REFERENCES

1. Uterus: definition - anatomy and functions (aly-abbara.com)

2. UTERUS (anat-jg.com)

3. anatomy-of-luterus.pdf (wordpress.com)

4. Hysterectomy - surgical and robotic expertise (gynecomarseille.com)

TECHNICAL SHEET: MACROSCOPIC MANAGEMENT OF PLACENTAS IN TWIN PREGNANCIES

GENERAL

■ Twin pregnancy is a pregnancy in which two foetuses develop in a single uterine cavity at the same time. It is also known as twin pregnancy, multiple pregnancy or multi-fetal pregnancy.

■ **Dizygotic twins (70%) = fraternal twins**

☐ Simultaneous fertilisation of 2 different oocytes, produced during the same menstrual cycle, by two different spermatozoa.

■ **Monozygotic twins (30%) = identical twins = identical genetic heritage**

☐ Division of a single fertilised egg (depending on the time between fertilisation and division of the fertilised egg, the type of placentation will be different).

■ Placenta examination is one of the diagnostic tools needed to explore any pathology in pregnancy or when an unusual aspect of the placenta is noted on ultrasound examination or in the delivery room at the time of delivery.

METHODOLOGY

A. Identification of the 2 twins :

- **For optimum examination: Each placenta must be identified for each twin.**
- This identification must be carried out in the delivery room, using a set of clamps on the cords for example (arrows).

- If this has not been done, an arbitrary identification will be made before the macroscopic examination begins.

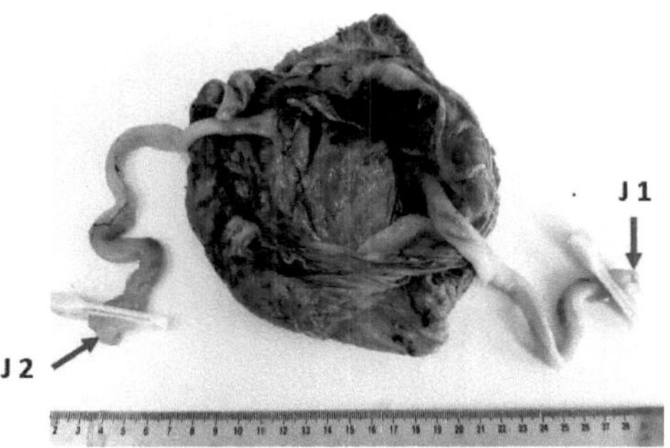

Figure 1: Identification of the 2 twins (J1 and J2) by a set of clamps on the cords (arrows).

B. Determining choriality :

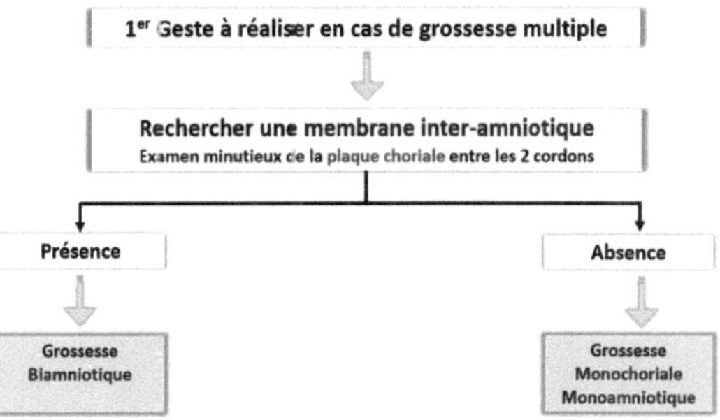

∎ In the case of a **bi-amniotic** pregnancy :

Aspect of the membrane :

☐ **Opaque, thick, cleavable:** probable **bichorionic pregnancy**
☐ **Translucent, thin, non-cleavable:** probable **monochorionic pregnancy**
(A definitive diagnosis can only be made by histological analysis)
 Removal of a strip of membrane (= 1 block)
☐ **2** to **3 mm** wide
☐ From placental insertion to the rupture zone
☐ Winding on Kocher forceps, taking care to place the end corresponding to the rupture zone
of the membranes in the centre of the coil.

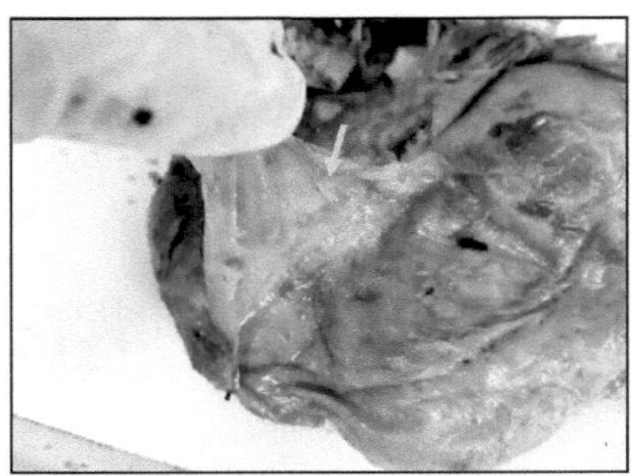

Figure 2: Macroscopic appearance of the inter-amniotic membrane (yellow arrow). It is opaque and thick.

C. Macroscopic examination :

1- Bichorionic biamniotic pregnancy with separate placentas :

Once the inter-amniotic membrane had been removed, the 2 placentas were examined separately as 2 placentas from singletons.

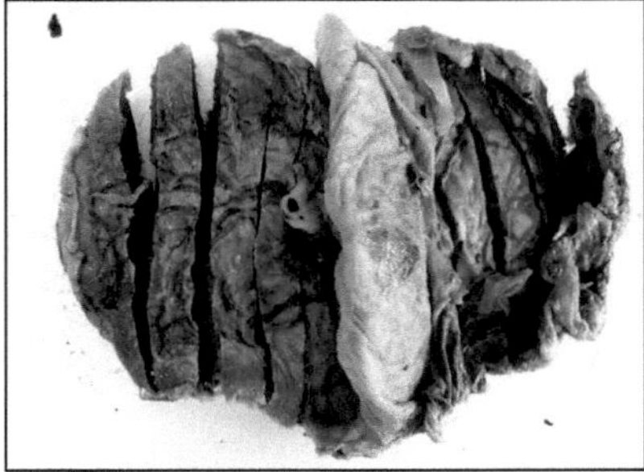

Figure 3: Serial slicing of the two placentas

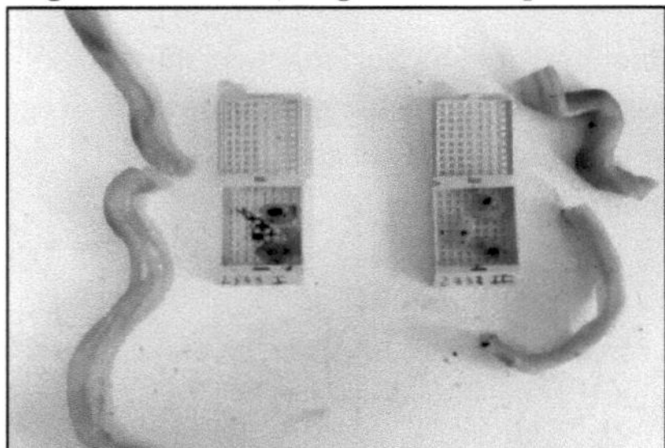

Figure 4: Samples taken from both umbilical cords

2. Bichorionic biamniotic pregnancy with fused placentas :

Examination of the umbilical cords
Each cord is examined separately:

- **Insertion:** The insertion of each is determined in relation to **the entire chorionic plate and not in relation to the inter-amniotic membrane.**

☐ **Measure the distance** between the bases of the 2 cords.

Examination of the placental disc
- After sectioning the entire placenta
- **Description** and **sampling of macroscopic lesions** and **any differences in appearance between the 2 areas (at least 3 blocks in each area** if there are no macroscopic lesions).

3. Monochorionic biamniotic pregnancy :
The macroscopic stages are **the same as for a single placenta**, with a few differences:

Inter-amniotic membrane

- Appearance, insertion on the chorionic plate

- **Sampling (= 1 block)**

Examination of the umbilical cords (each cord is examined separately)

- **Insertion:** the insertion of each of the cords is determined in relation to **the entire chorionic plate and not in relation to the inter-amniotic membrane.**
- **Measuring the distance** between the bases of the 2 cords

Examination of the chorionic plate
Examination **of the arborisation of the allanto-chorionic vessels is essential:**

- Assessment of the respective vascular territories.
- Search for **superficial vascular anastomoses** (without pathological consequences).
- Search for possible starting points **of deep arteriovenous anastomoses** (difficult to detect on macro examination) (= risk of transfusion-transfusion syndrome)

Creation of sectional slices of the entire placental disc
☐ Parenchyma thickness and colour
☐ **Description and sampling of macroscopic lesions** and **any differences in appearance between the 2 areas (at least 3 blocks in each area** if there are no macroscopic lesions).

2- Monochorionic monoamniotic pregnancy

The macroscopic stages are **the same as for a single placenta,** with a few differences.

Examination of the umbilical cords
(Each cord is examined separately)

☐ **Insertion:** the insertion of each of the cords is determined by reference to **the entire chorionic plate.**
- **measure the distance** between the bases of the 2 cords
Examination of the chorionic plate

Examination **of the arborisation of the allanto-chorionic vessels :**
▪ Assessment of the respective vascular territories
▪ **Search for vascular anastomoses (constant in monochorionic monoamniotic pregnancies)**

Creation of sectional slices of the entire placental disc
▪ Parenchyma thickness and colour

▪ **Staged sampling of macroscopically healthy areas and sampling of macroscopic lesions (at least 4 blocks if no macroscopic lesions)**

What to sample

☐ **Biamniotic pregnancies (mono or bichorionic)**

Systematic sampling

☐ The **inter-amniotic membrane** (1 block)

☐ A **ribbon of membranes** and **2 sections of cord** for each twin

→ At least **3 macroscopically healthy blocks of placenta in each territory**

→ Sampling **of macroscopic lesions** and any difference in appearance between the **territories of** the 2 twins

Monochorionic monoamniotic pregnancy
☐
Systematic sampling

☐ 2 sections of cord for each twin

☐ A **ribbon of membranes**

→ At least **4 blocks of placenta in macroscopically healthy areas and macroscopic lesions**

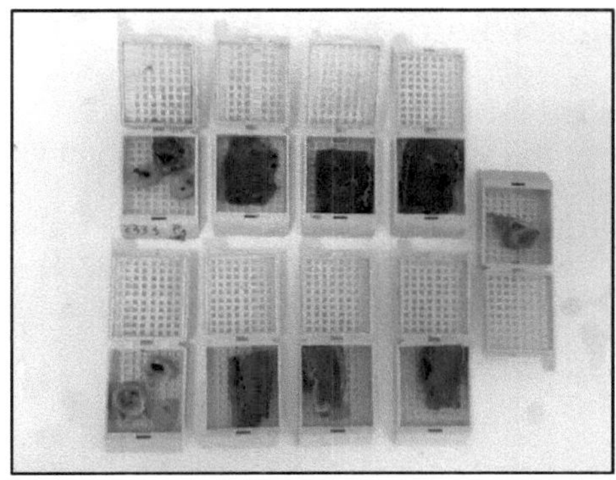

Figure 5: samples taken from the placentas of a bichorionic biamniotic pregnancy with separate placentas are placed in cassettes.

MATERIAL REQUIRED

29. **Fixing agent:** The usual fixing agent is 10% buffered formalin.
30. **Scalpel blade - knife**
31. **Flat ruler**
32. **Cassettes**
33. **Tape measure**
34. **Camera**

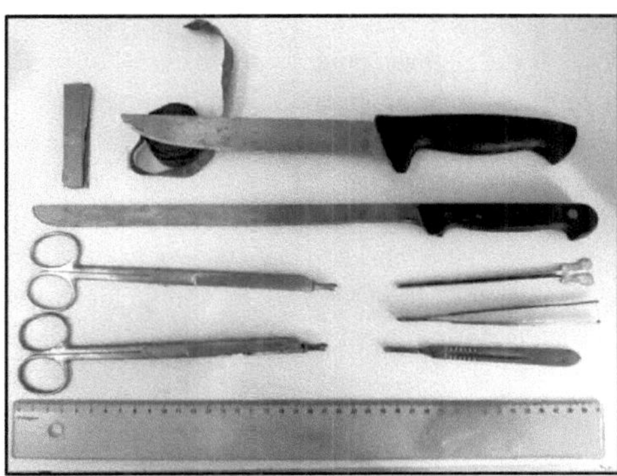

Figure 6: Equipment required for macroscopic examination

CONDITIONS AND RULES OF GOOD PRACTICE

▪ Placentas are fixed for 24 - 48 hours in 10% buffered formalin.
▪ Delayed or poor fixation will affect the morphological quality of the histological sections. Respect the ratio of tissue volume to fixative volume (1/10).
▪ All placental specimens must be sent to the pathological anatomy laboratory with a clinical information sheet describing the history of the disease, the mother's history, the course of the pregnancy, the results of the paraclinical examinations carried out and the treatment administered.

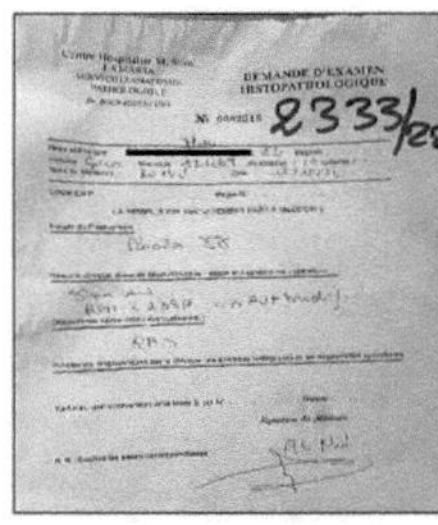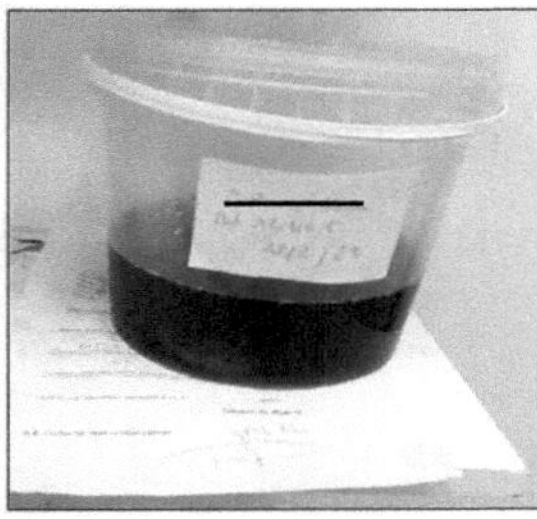

Figure 7: Clinical information sheet accompanying placental specimens from twin pregnancies sent to the pathology laboratory.

CONCLUSION

▪ The placenta, which bears witness to intrauterine life, should be sent to the pathological anatomy laboratory if there is the slightest doubt about maternal or foetal pathology, or if the placenta is abnormal, together with the essential clinical information.
▪ In the specific case of the death of a child, whether in utero or in the immediate post-partum period, the placenta must be examined along with the foetus as part of a complete foetopathological examination. This is a simple, low-cost procedure, requiring the standard equipment found in all pathology laboratories.
▪ Analysis of the lesions enables the child or mother to be monitored or treated appropriately, depending on the case, or attempts to prevent recurrence of the lesions in subsequent pregnancies.

REFERENCES

1. Cornélis F. The value of anatomopathological examination of the placenta. Revue Francophone des laboratoires 2008; 402: 71-76.
2. Hargitai B., Marton T., Cox P.M., Best practice no 178, Examination of the human placenta, J Clin Pathol 2004; 57: 785-792.
3. Nessmann C., Larroche J.C., Atlas de pathologie placentaire, Masson, 2001, p 22-24.

TECHNICAL SHEET: MACROSCOPIC MANAGEMENT OF MASTECTOMY PARTS

ANATOMICAL OVERVIEW OF THE BREAST

The breast can be divided into regions:

- **the central region** corresponding to the area behind the nipple
- **4 quadrants** located on either side of a cross made up of 2 perpendicular segments whose intersection is at the level of the nipple: superior-internal quadrant (QSI), superior-external quadrant (QSE), infero-external quadrant (QIE) and inferointernal quadrant (QII).

There are also :

- **Axillary extension**: territory located in the extension of the external quadrants towards the axillary hollow
- **The sub-mammary fold**: an area located at the boundary between the lower quadrants and the chest wall

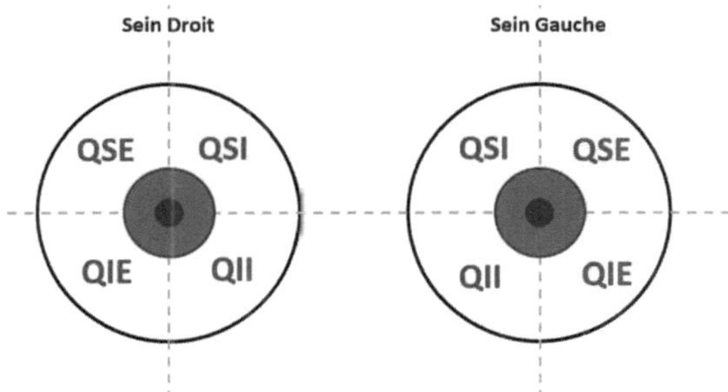

Fig.1 : Subdivision of the right and left breast into 4 quadrants

METHODOLOGY

GUIDANCE

Simple mastectomy
This sample includes :
- the **mammary gland**
- the **skin** covering it
- the **nipple-areolar plate**

- possibly a **fragment of the** pectoralis major **muscle**, in the case of a deep tumour.

It is important to know the side of the breast. The surgeon can put 2 marks on the skin: notches, sutures, staples: 1 on the upper side and 1 on the inner side, for example.

Mastectomy with conservation of the skin covering after diagnosis of ductal carcinoma in situ on macrobiopsy.

This sample includes :
- the **mammary gland**
- the **nipple-areolar plate**.
It is important to know the side of the breast. The surgeon can place 2 markers on the nipple-areolar plate: notches, sutures, staples: 1 on the upper side and 1 on the inner side, for example.
It is imperative that an **X-ray of the surgical specimen** is sent to the pathologist, who must mention it in his report.

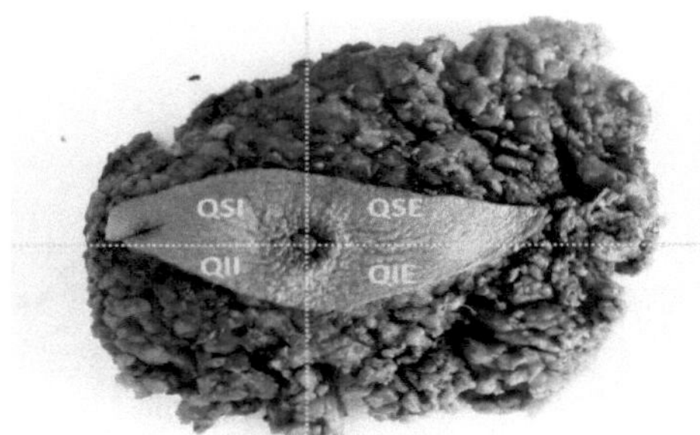

Fig. 2: Left mastectomy with an internal marker (internal wire).

ENCRAGE

▪ **Simple mastectomy :**

In general, it is not necessary to ink this sample, unless the lesion is close to one of the resection margins, particularly the deep margin. In this case, the deep margin should be inked.

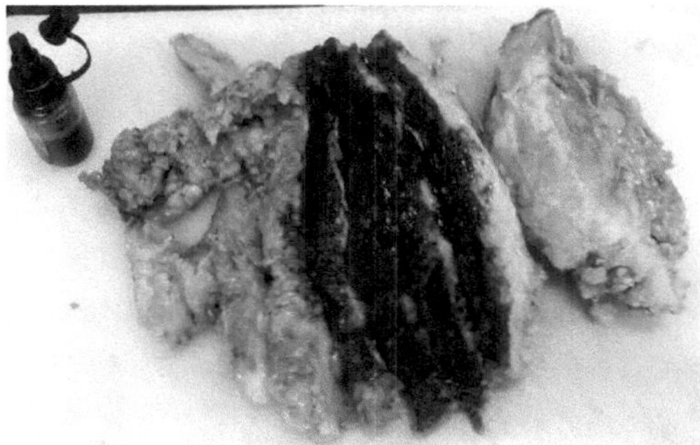

Fig. 3: Inking of the deep plane of a mastectomy part

- **Mastectomy with preservation of the skin cover :**

This sample is generally taken for extensive ISCC (In-Situ Ductal Carcinoma).
You need to ink the surface of the bank one colour and the deep bank a different colour.

PART MEASUREMENT

This stage consists of **measuring the mastectomy** in the three planes of space as well as
the adjoining **skin flap** or nipple-areolar plate.

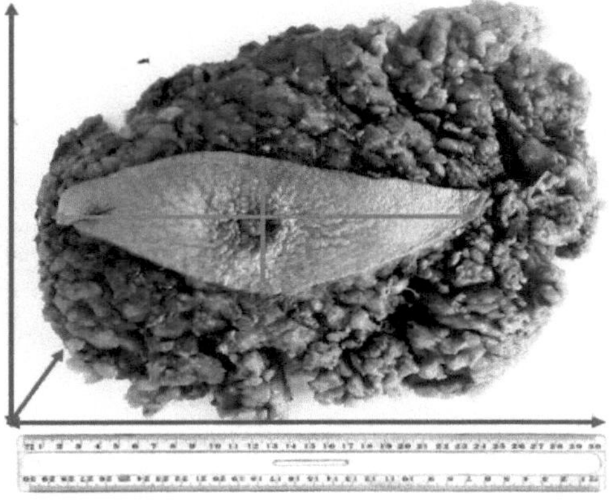

Fig.4. Measurements of a mastectomy specimen

PRE-CUTTING THE PART

• Simple mastectomy

Slice the mastectomy posteriorly, preserving the integrity of the skin covering (book-leaf slices). It is preferable to carry out this step in the fresh state, as pre-cutting the mastectomy makes it easier to fix.

• Mastectomy with preservation of the skin cover

As these surgical parts are often thin, it is not necessary to slice them. If it is nevertheless necessary, take care to leave the slices joined together so as not to lose the markings. Leave the nipple-areolar plate in place

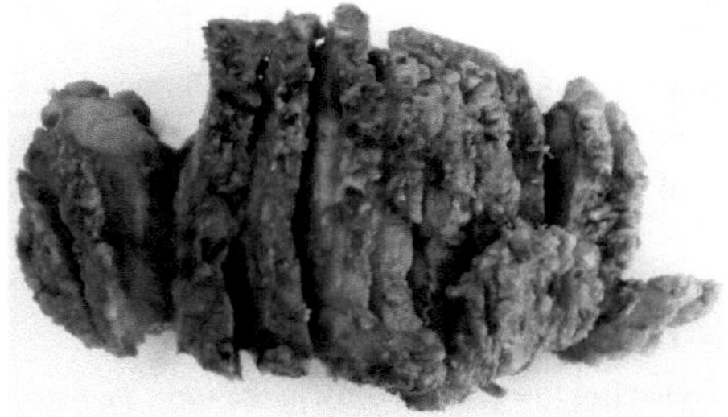

Fig.5: Slicing the mastectomy posteriorly to form a book leaf.

IDENTIFYING AND DESCRIBING LESIONS

✓ **Locate the nodule(s) by sight or palpation.**

Palpation is particularly useful on a fresh specimen and can be used to adjust the size of a tumour. A tumour may be more palpable than visible (infiltrating lobular carcinoma).

✓ **Note** their location (quadrant) and their distance from the resection margins.
✓ **Open** the nodule(s) along its/their longest axis and in the middle.

✓ **Measure the largest diameter of the tumour(s)**

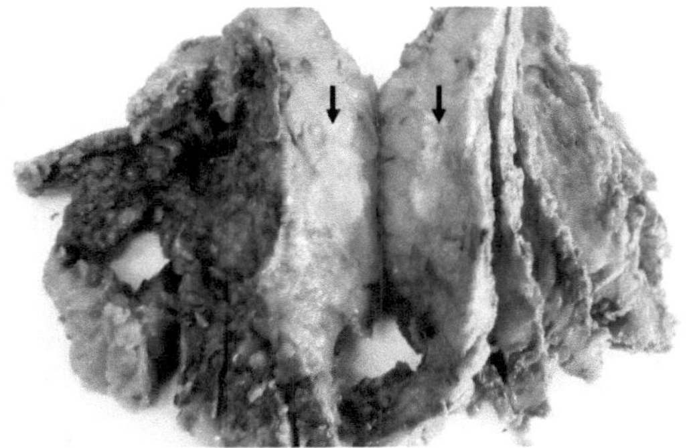

Fig.6 : Location of the tumour lesion (arrows) in the mastectomy specimen

PRE-CUT NIPPLE

Simple mastectomy

Remove the nipple: to do this, lay the part flat, posterior side down on the macroscopy board and pull the nipple upwards using forceps. Cut deeply into the nipple with a scalpel, following the contour of the areola. Leave some breast tissue next to the nipple. This step is important so that the nipple can be analysed separately and to allow optimal fixation of the mastectomy.

Mastectomy with preservation of the skin cover

Leave the nipple and areola in place on the part before fixing.

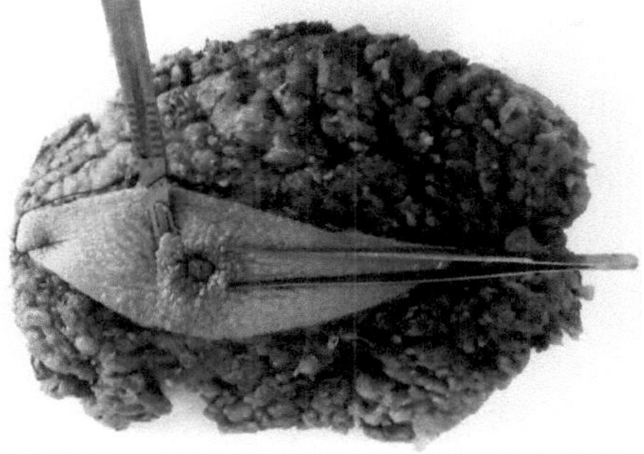

Fig.7. Pre-cutting the nipple using claw forceps and a scalpel blade

SYSTEMATIC SAMPLING

▪ **Nipple**: 2-3 samples taken perpendicular to the skin plane, 1 retromammary sample taken parallel to the skin plane

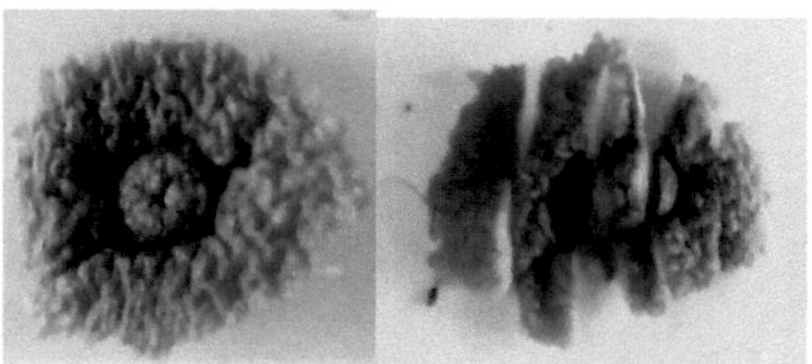

Fig.8: samples taken perpendicular to the skin of the nipple

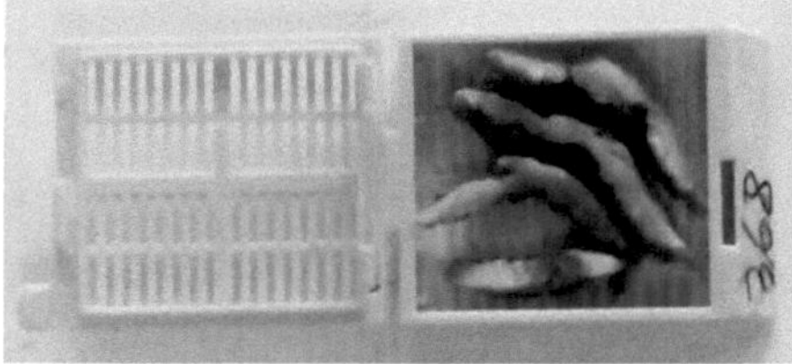

Fig.9 : Putting the samples taken from the nipple into a plastic cassette

▪ **Other quadrants:** in invasive cancers, samples are not systematically taken as they have no therapeutic impact, unless macroscopic lesions are present.

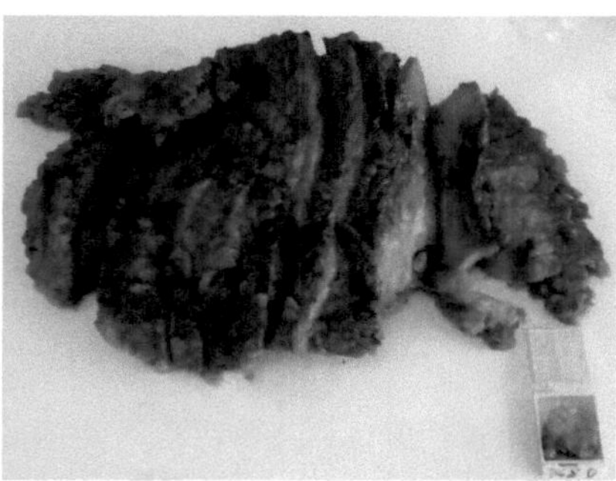

Fig.10: Systematic sampling of the lower medial quadrant of the left breast

SAMPLING THE TUMOUR

Locatable tumour

‾ A minimum of **3 samples**, including a representative section of the tumour in its longest axis.

‾ **In the case of a deep tumour,** in contact with the pectoral, mark the **boundary** and remove it.

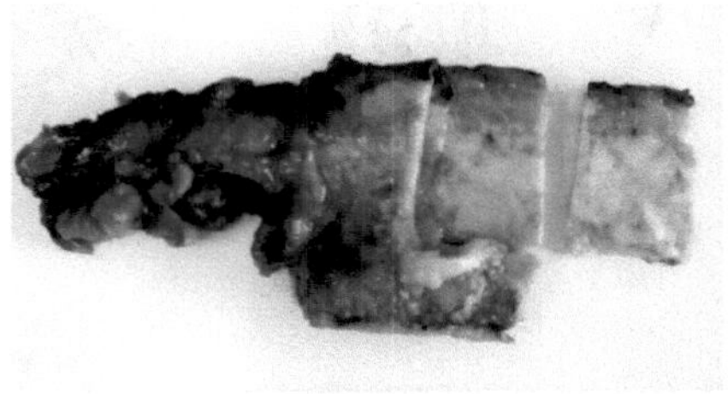

Fig. 11: Sample taken from within the tumour

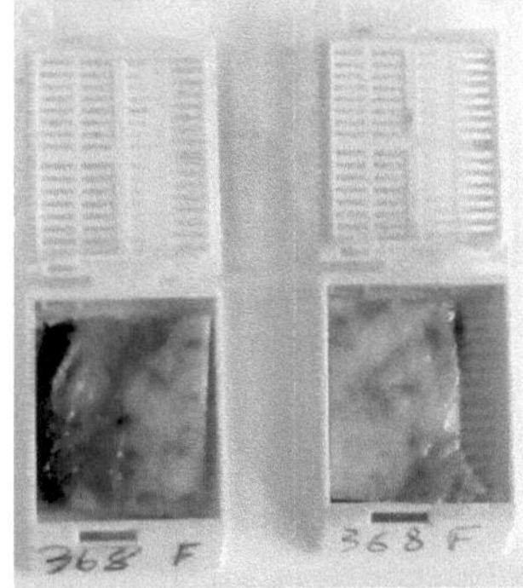

Fig.12 : Putting tumour samples in a plastic cassette

AXILLARY RECURRENCE

All lymph nodes are sampled and included in their entirety

• Each lymph node is included in a cassette and identified as G1, G2, G3, G4 ... (one node per number)

• The largest lymph nodes are cut into serial macroscopic slices 2 mm thick. If a lymph node is divided into several cassettes, label them G1A, G1B...

• A representative section is sufficient for lymph nodes that are clearly invaded on macroscopic examination.

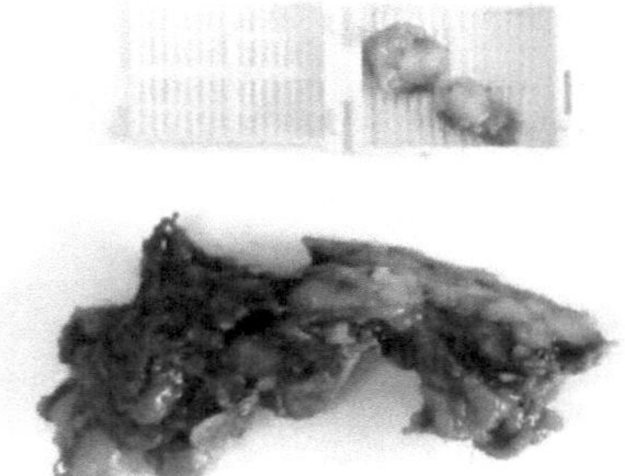

Fig. 13 : Lymph node dissection

It is desirable to examine a minimum of 6 lymph nodes for pTNM staging, but it is recommended to examine a minimum of 10 nodes per curage for valid prognostic information.

MATERIAL REQUIRED

• **Fixing agent:** The usual fixing agent is 10% buffered formalin.
• **Scalpel blade - knife**
• **Cassettes**
• **Camera**

CONDITIONS AND RULES OF GOOD PRACTICE

Delayed or poor fixation will adversely affect the morphological quality of histological sections. Respect the ratio between the quantity of tissue and the volume of fixative (1/10).

CONCLUSION

The aim of macroscopic examination of breast excision specimens is to obtain information about the morphological, topographical and histopronostic aspects that are useful for diagnosing and treating breast lesions. It determines the subsequent microscopic analysis. Management must take account of clinical and mammographic information. The possibility of neoadjuvant treatment must be specified. In the case of surgical specimens, the type of surgical excision carried out must be specified in order to assess them correctly.

TECHNICAL SHEET: MACROSCOPIC MANAGEMENT OF A CONE SECTION

• **Target audience**: residents in pathological anatomy
• **Prepared by** : Dr Faten LIMAIEM

ANATOMY OF THE UTERINE CERVIX - GENERAL INFORMATION

■ **The wall of the uterine cervix is formed by :**

- A fibromuscular wall in continuity with the uterine myometrium
- In contact with light :
▪ The endocervix below t h e isthmus and endometrium, opposite the
cervical canal
▪ The ectocervix is opposite the vaginal cavity. It is bounded laterally by
through the right and left paracervix (not peritonealised)

■ **Conization :**
Conization: is the removal of part of the cervix (the peri-orificial pathological zone). It can be performed using a cold knife, laser or, more often, a diathermic loop. It is recommended in cases of cellular changes (dysplasia) of the cervix diagnosed by smear and confirmed by colposcopy and biopsy. If left untreated, these lesions can develop into cervical cancer after several years. The aim of the operation is twofold: to confirm the exact extent and type of dysplasia, and in the majority of cases to remove the lesions completely, thereby preventing progression to cancer.

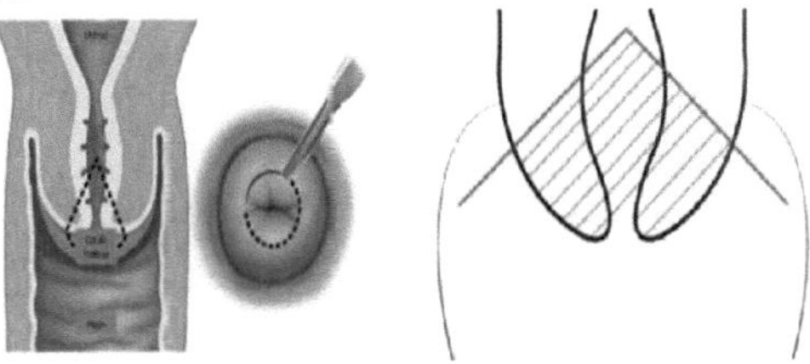

Figure 1: Conization
Figure 2: conization
www.paptestinfo.ca/includes/panel4_f.html Pelvic surgery - Gynéco Cannes
(gynecocannes.com)

METHODOLOGY

1. Orientation :

The part must be marked out by the surgeon using a marker wire or an incision, usually at 12 o'clock.

The exocervical epithelium has a pearly white appearance and the endocervical epithelium contains mucus.

2. Description of the operating room :
- Specify whether the surgical specimen is **fresh** or **fixed**
- Specify the **fixative** used
- Specify whether the item was received closed or open
- Size :
- **Width**mm
- **Height**mm
- **Thickness**mm

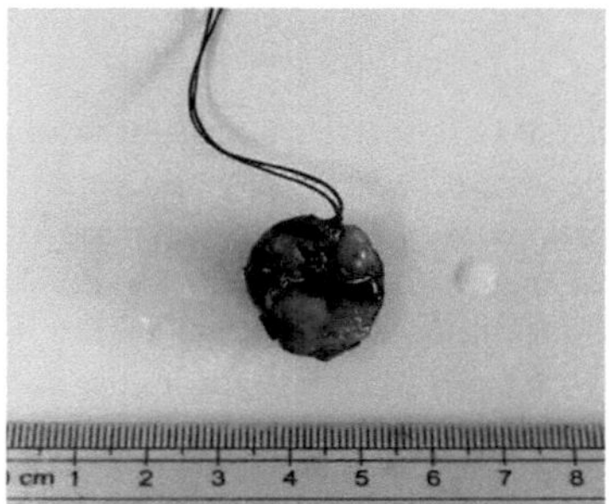

Figure 3: Conization piece oriented by a 12 o'clock wire

3. Inking (optional) and part opening :
- Optional inking :
- **Front side**
- **Posterior side**
- If the cervix is closed, gently insert a fine cannula and open at 12 o'clock.

4. Describe the lesion :
- Lesion: assessable / not assessable
- Macroscopic appearance :
- **Ulcerative**

- **Plant**
- **Infiltrant**
- **Well limited**
- **Badly limited**

  -Measurements: surface size: ... X ... mm

Infiltration depth: ... mm (to be measured after cutting)

5. Serial macroscopic sections of a conization

- Serial macroscopic slices with a thickness of 2 - 3 mm are included in their **entirety.**

- Put one macroscopic slice per cassette and do not include the same mirror face on two slices.

c. First Method:

Closed neck: radial sections; clockwise/counterclockwise inclusion

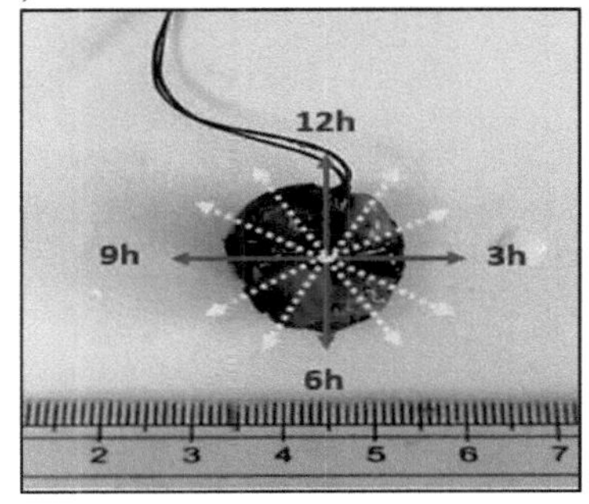

b. Second Method: Inclusion in the sense :

→ From right to left

→ From left to right

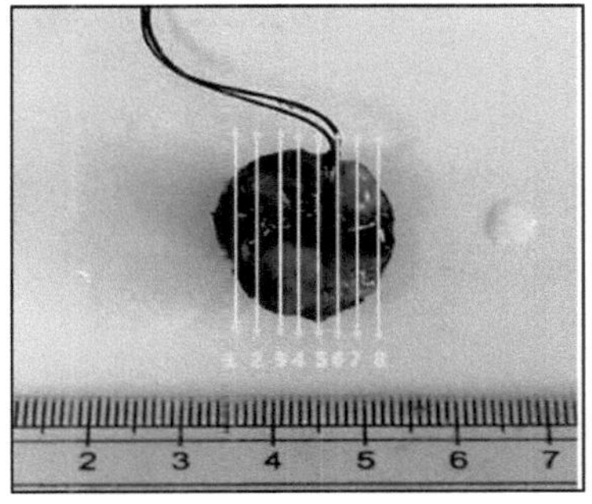

c. Third Method: Open and spread collar :

- Clockwise / anti-clockwise inclusion
- Locate the reference of the blocks at the cardinal points (12h, 3h, 6h, 9h).
-

MATERIAL REQUIRED
- **Fixing agent:** The usual fixing agent is 10% buffered formalin.
- **Scalpel blade**
- **Cassettes**
- **Camera**

CONDITIONS AND RULES OF GOOD PRACTICE

- The surgical specimen is fixed for 24 hours in formalin.
10% buffered.

- Delayed or poor fixation will affect the morphological quality of the histological sections. Respect the ratio of tissue volume to fixative volume (1/10).

CONCLUSION
- Macroscopic examination of conization specimens contributes to patient management by assessing prognosis and defining important criteria for prescribing any additional post-operative treatment.

REFERENCES
10. Conisation.pdf (hug.ch)

11. Jean-Charles Boulanger, Jean Gondry, Philippe Naepels. Conisations. EMC Techniques chirurgicales. [41-685]

TECHNICAL SHEET: PREPARATION OF CERVICO-VAGINAL SMEAR SLIDES

DEFINITION

• Cytological analysis of gynaecological specimens aims to reveal the presence of abnormal or cancerous cells by performing a microscopic analysis of the cells of the uterine cervix. This analysis enables early detection of cervical cancer, thereby helping to reduce the incidence of mortality due to this type of cancer.

• Cytological analysis can also detect non-specific hormonal changes, as well as the presence of certain parasites, viruses or fungi.

GYNAECOLOGICAL SAMPLING: METHODOLOGY

1. Direct debit :

1.1. Levy from ectocervix and of the endocervical junction

It is performed using the rounded end of the Ayre spatula, the special shape of which allows elements of the endovaginal part of the ectocervix to be scraped off and, above all, the cells of the junction zone between the squamous squamous epithelium of the ectocervix and the cylindrical glandular epithelium of the endocervix, the birthplace of cervical dysplasia, to be obtained.
This zone is located at the circular boundary between the smooth, pinkish exocervical surface and the more granular periorificial red zone (this marker is approximate; it can be seen more accurately on colposcopy after the application of acetic acid).
The tapered end of the Ayre spatula is positioned in contact with the external cervical os and, using a rotary movement, the entire junction area is swept concentrically.

The cell material collected at the end of the spatula is then spread onto a first glass slide, avoiding repeating the process in the same place to ensure that the cells spread evenly. The cells are immediately fixed using a spray (hairspray), sprayed perpendicular to the slide from a distance of around twenty centimetres to avoid the cells becoming detached.

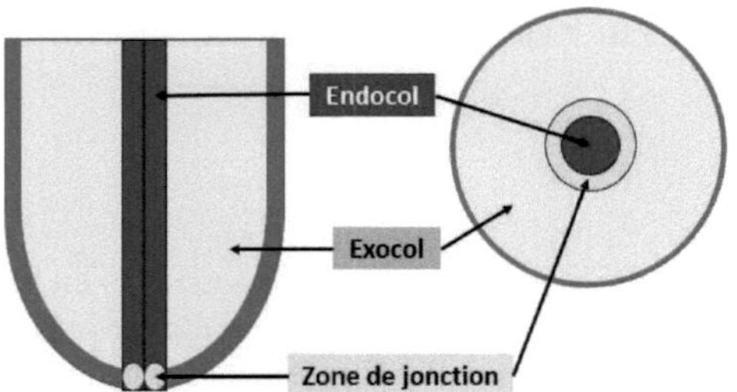

Fig 1: Areas where cervico-vaginal smears are taken

1.2. Endocervical sampling :

A swab or cytobrush is inserted into the first centimetre of the endocervical canal and, by moving back and forth inside the endocervix, the glandular cells and endocervical mucus are collected. The juice collected on the swab is rolled out in several lines over the entire surface of a second slide.

The spread must be regular, linear and continuous. A thin layer of cells must be produced without crushing them. In this way, the cells are found in a trail and in single file, which makes it easier to interpret the smear. Fixation must also be immediate. Brush smears are not systematically recommended as they are often more haemorrhagic.

2. Spreading :

Using an Ayre spatula, mounted rod or cytobrush, spread the specimen as evenly as possible by exerting gentle pressure on the slide. The spreading movement should be linear in order to keep the abnormal cells in the adjacent microscopic fields for better detection. The spread should be neither too thin because of the risk of obtaining an unrepresentative specimen nor too thick because of the risk of masking abnormal cells.

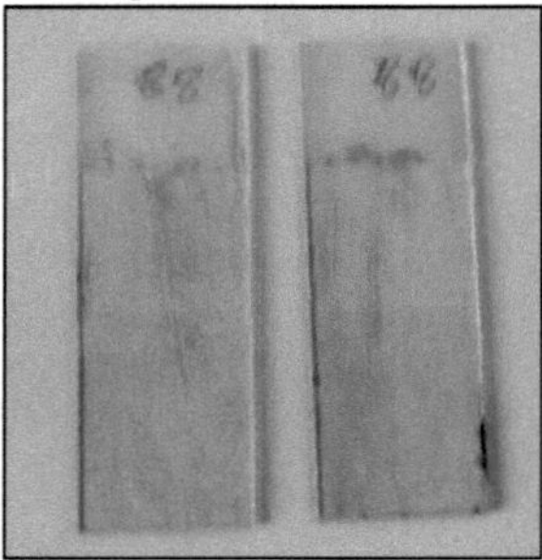

Fig 2: Spreading on a slide of samples taken from the endocervix and the the ectocervix

3. Mounting :

• Fix the smear immediately after spreading using an aerosol fixative;
• Keep the fixative at a distance of about 15 to 20 cm from the slide;
a. A closer distance runs the risk of damaging the cells or creating artefacts ;
b. A greater distance may not adequately cover the cells.
• Leave to dry for at least 10 minutes;
• Store slides at room temperature, in a container that protects them from external contaminants.

4. Packaging and transport :

• Place each of the clearly labelled slides in a carton or transport box;
• Attach the corresponding requests;
• Send specimens and requests to the cytology laboratory.

5. Colouring with Papanicolaou :

Papanicolaou" staining is the globally adopted staining method for cytological specimens. It is polychromatic, since it contains a nuclear dye.

Papanicolaou dye is composed of three dyes:

• **Harris** haematoxylin: stains cell nuclei thanks to its affinity with DNA.
• Orange G **(OG 6)**: reacts with mature squamous cells due to its affinity with keratin.

• Eosin-azur **(EA 50)**: reacts with the cytoplasm of non-mature squamous cells (basal and intermediate cells) as well as glandular cells and red blood cells.
Nuclear staining may be progressive or regressive. The choice of method used depends on the results obtained and the personal preferences of the pathologist and/or cytologists.

• **Progressive method**: Continuous colouring until the desired intensity is achieved;

• **Regressive method**: The specimen is over-coloured in haematoxylin, then the excess dye is removed by immersion in a differentiator (0.25% HCL (hydrochloric acid)). Immersion under running water then stops the chemical discolouration reaction.

5.1. Preparing the "Papanicolaou" colouring

1. Filter all the dyes used;
2. Mix the dye well in the bottle before use;
3. In a fume cupboard, prepare the alcohol solutions at the required percentages (50%, 70%,

80%, 95% and 100%);

4) Under a chemical hood, filter and/or fill the solvent baths (xylene and/or toluene);

5) Always under the chemical hood:

a. If the progressive method is used: Add 4% acetic acid to Harris haematoxylin;

b. If the regressive method is used: Prepare the 0.25% HCL bath.

6) Position the baths according to the chosen method;

7) Put the lids on the baths and remove them just before colouring.

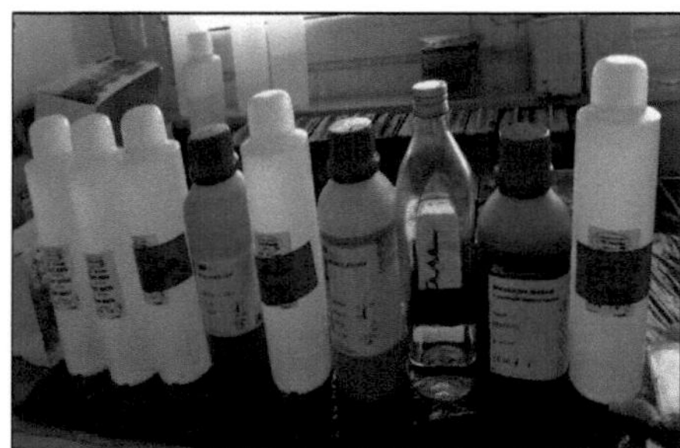

Fig. 3: Different products used for Papanicolaou staining

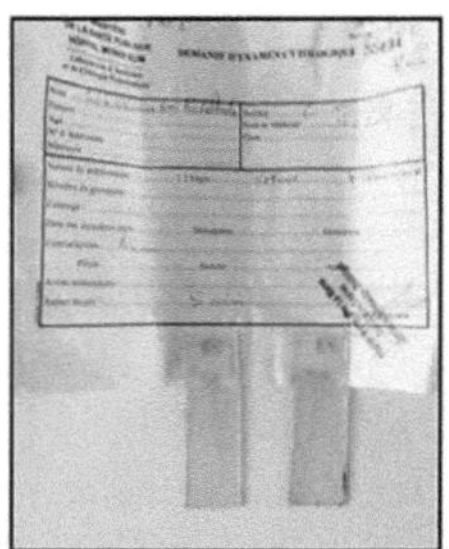

Fig.4. Frottis cervico-vaginal accompagné d'une fiche de renseignements cliniques

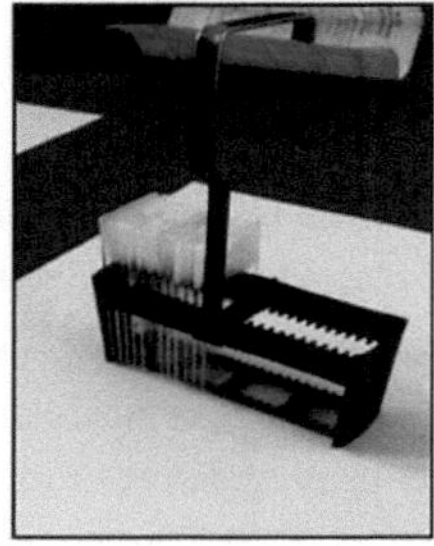

Fig.5. L'ensemble des lames est mis dans un portoir

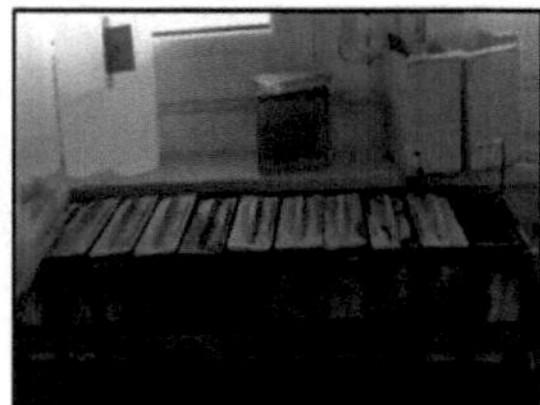

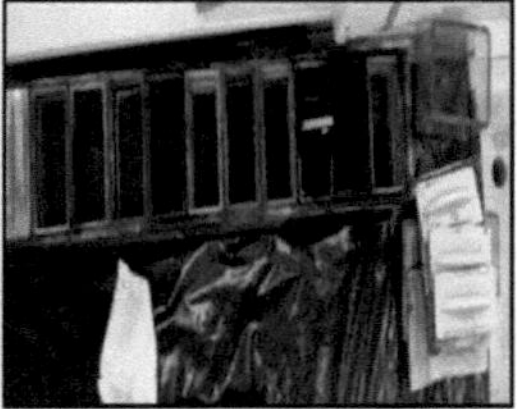

Fig.6. Différents bains contenant les solutions nécessaires pour la coloration Papanicolaou

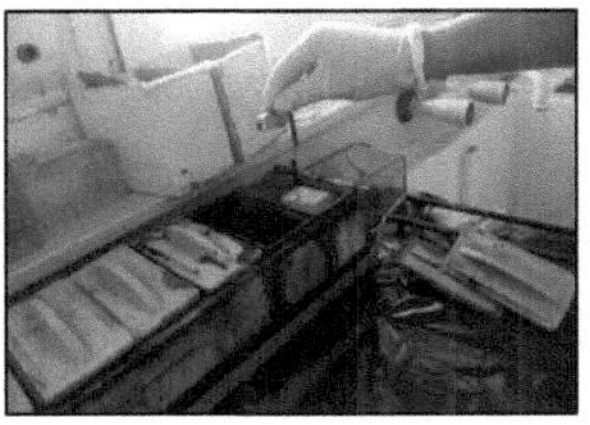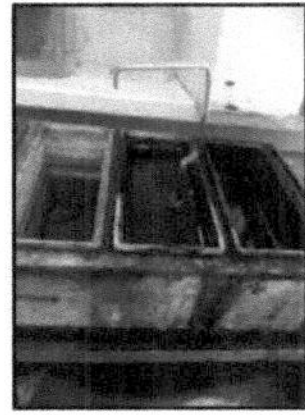

Fig. 7. : Le portoir de lames de FCU est plongé successivement dans les différents bains contenant les solutions nécessaires pour la coloration Papanicolaou

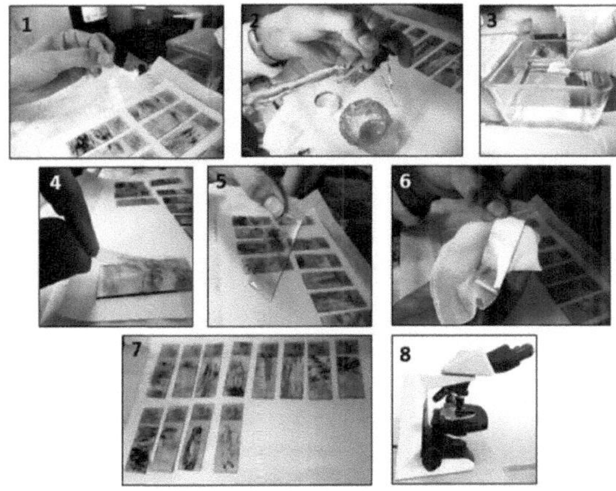

Fig.8: Different stages of slide mounting (1-6), followed by reading of the slides under an optical microscope.

5.2. Results :

• Cell nuclei are stained blue/black
• The cytoplasm of keratinised cells is pink/transparent orange (depending on the concentration of ethanol in the stain).
• The cytoplasm of non-keratinised cells is in transparent blue/green.
• Red blood cells are in red

6. Gynaecological sampling in liquid medium

Cervical cells are collected using the same methods as for conventional smears. Once the cervix has been visualised using the speculum, a sample is taken using a brush specifically designed for liquid-based cytology. The brush is then placed in a liquid fixative. Suspension in the liquid ensures complete release of the cells. Depending on the equipment chosen by the laboratory, the sample processing methods may differ. The thin-film technique removes some of the mucus and inflammatory cells.

The main advantages of this method are
- The samples of cells taken are more representative and the cells are better preserved;
- Increased detection of intraepithelial lesions;
- The reading time required is shortened;
- Additional smears can be taken from the same sample;
- A reduction in the diagnosis of ASC-US and AGC;
- The possibility of using complementary techniques, such as

HPV testing and typing, immunocytochemistry

MATERIALS REQUIRED FOR PAPANICOLAOU COLOURING

1. ALCOHOL 95

To obtain 500 ml of 95% alcohol, mix :

- 475 ml absolute ethyl alcohol ;
- 25 ml water (distilled).

2. ALCOHOL 80

To obtain 500 ml of 80% alcohol, mix :

- 400 ml absolute ethyl alcohol ;
- 100 ml water (distilled).

3. 70% ALCOHOL

To obtain 500 ml of 70% alcohol, mix :

- 350 ml absolute ethyl alcohol ;
- 150 ml water (distilled).

4. **ALCOHOL 50%** To obtain 500 ml of alcohol 50%, mix :

- 250 ml absolute ethyl alcohol ;
- 250 ml water (distilled).

5. **ALCOHOL-XYLENE (OR TOLUENE)**
To obtain 500 ml of xylene alcohol (or toluene), mix :
- 250 ml absolute ethyl alcohol ;
- 250 ml xylene (or toluene).

6. **HCL AT 0.25%**
To obtain 400 ml of 0.25% hydrochloric acid, mix :
- 399 ml water (distilled) ;
- 1 ml HCl.

7. **NH4OH AT 1.5**
To obtain 400 ml of ammonium hydroxide (or ammonia water), mix :
- 394 ml 70% alcohol;
- 6 ml ammonium hydroxide (NH4OH).

COLOUR QUALITY ASSESSMENT

Staining quality should be assessed after each staining sequence and documented.

Table 1: Evaluation of "Papanicolaou" colouring

Dyes and expected colour	Standards
Haematoxylin Nuclei: blue or dark purple	The nuclear outline is well defined and its colour contrasts with the cytoplasmic staining; The chromatin is clearly visible; The interlobular links of the polynuclear cells are visible.
OG6 Squames: orange-yellow Keratinised cells: bright orange	The orange colour is not usually visible in a normal smear, unless scales are present.
EA (36, 50 or 65) Superficial cells: pink Intermediate cells: blue Parabasal cells: bright blue-green	The cytoplasm of each cell must be translucent; The nuclei and cytoplasmic outlines of cells in clusters are clearly visible through the cytoplasm.

RECOMMENDATIONS

• To optimise specimen staining, it is recommended that the slides are immersed in 95% alcohol for approximately 20 minutes before staining. This immersion allows the fixatives present on the slides to be cleaned (especially if an aerosol fixative has been used) and the effects of the stains used to be optimised.

• While it is recommended that all staining baths be installed under a chemical hood when staining is carried out manually, it is advisable to use lukewarm running water during automated staining.

CONCLUSION

In conclusion, the "Practical Guide to Macroscopy in Pathological Anatomy - Essential Guidelines" is much more than just a manual; it is an indispensable companion in the complex world of surgical specimen analysis. Through precise guidelines and rigorous protocols, this guide lights the way for anatomopathologists, helping them to decode the mysteries buried in every tissue examined. Macroscopic examination is an essential starting point, revealing crucial information for the diagnosis, prognosis and treatment of pathological conditions. From meticulous fixation to meticulous inclusion, each stage of this process requires special attention and expert know-how to guarantee reliable and significant results.By embracing the complexity of the tissues examined, navigating the nuances of lesions and interpreting the clues left in each specimen, pathologists continue to be the guardians of diagnostic accuracy and quality patient care. This guide, with its essential role in the practice of pathological anatomy, remains a fundamental pillar for all those engaged in the quest to understand and solve medical enigmas. Through its diligent and respectful use of established protocols, it contributes tirelessly to the advancement of medical science and the well-being of patients throughout the world.

REFERENCES

1) Fetal autopsy: a relevant medical procedure | Documents de Médecine Légale (wordpress.com)

2) Kalousek DK. Pathology of abortion: the embryo and the previable fetus. In Gilbert-Barness E (ed.). Potter's pathology of the fetus and infant. St. Louis: Mosby; 1997.p. 106.

3) Emmrich P, Horn LC, Seifert U. [Morphologic findings in fetuses and placentas of late abortion in the 2nd trimester]. Zentralbl Gynakol. 1998;120(8):399-405.

4) Marton T, Hargitai B, Patkós P, Csapó Z, Szende B, Papp Z. [Practice of fetal pathological examination]. [Practice of fetal pathological examination. Orv Hetil. 1999 Jun 20;140(25):1411-6.

5) Pathologic Examination of Fetal and Placental Tissue Obtained by Dilation and Evacuation | Archives of Pathology & Laboratory Medicine | Allen Press

6) Item.pdf (lsmuni.lt)

7) course.pdf (confkhalifa.com)

8) The-Ovaries.pdf (uca.ma)

9) Uterine-Tromps.pdf (uca.ma)

10) UTERINE TRUMPS (univ-batna2.dz)

11) Uterus: definition - anatomy and functions (aly-abbara.com)

12) UTERUS (anat-jg.com)

13) anatomy-of-luterus.pdf (wordpress.com)

14) Hysterectomy - surgical and robotic expertise (gynecomarseille.com)

15) Cornélis F. The value of anatomopathological examination of the placenta. Revue Francophone des laboratoires 2008; 402: 71-76.

16) Hargitai B., Marton T., Cox P.M., Best practice no 178, Examination of the human placenta, J Clin Pathol 2004; 57: 785-792.

17) Nessmann C., Larroche J.C., Atlas de pathologie placentaire, Masson, 2001, p 22- 24.

18) Conisation.pdf (hug.ch)

19) Jean-Charles Boulanger,Jean Gondry,Philippe Naepels.Conisations.EMCTechniques chirurgicales. [41-685]

SUMMARY

This comprehensive guide to medical macroscopy offers an in-depth exploration of the various gynaecological pathologies, from myomas to adnexectomies and cystectomies. It also covers specific cases, such as the non-tumorous uterus and the particularities of placentas in twin pregnancies, as well as procedures such as mastectomy, conisation and cervico-uterine smear analysis. Each section details the essential protocols for the macroscopic examination of surgical specimens associated with these pathologies. This manual is designed to guide healthcare professionals in the rigorous analysis of specimens, thereby promoting accurate diagnoses and appropriate patient management.

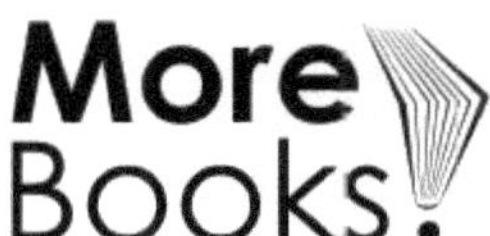
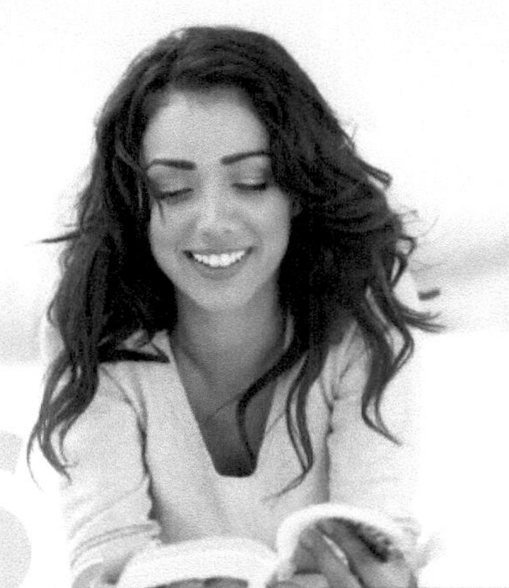

I want morebooks!

Buy your books fast and straightforward online - at one of world's fastest growing online book stores! Environmentally sound due to Print-on-Demand technologies.

Buy your books online at
www.morebooks.shop

Kaufen Sie Ihre Bücher schnell und unkompliziert online – auf einer der am schnellsten wachsenden Buchhandelsplattformen weltweit! Dank Print-On-Demand umwelt- und ressourcenschonend produziert.

Bücher schneller online kaufen
www.morebooks.shop

info@omniscriptum.com
www.omniscriptum.com

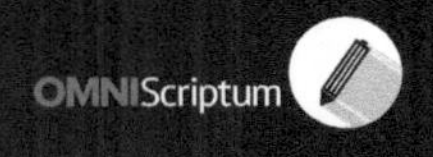

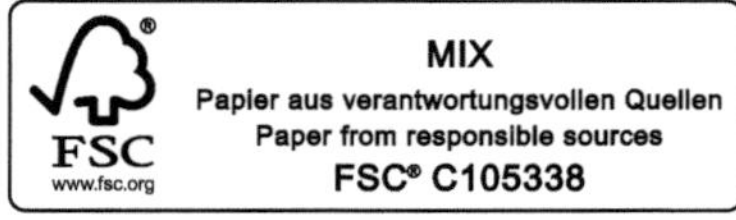

Printed by Books on Demand GmbH, Norderstedt / Germany